Donated by Highlands Cashiers Health Foundation

WORLD OF DRONES

Medical DRONES

Bradley Steffens

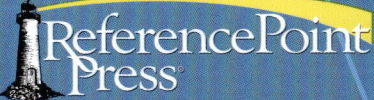

San Diego, CA

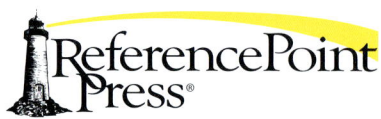

© 2021 ReferencePoint Press, Inc.
Printed in the United States

For more information, contact:
ReferencePoint Press, Inc.
PO Box 27779
San Diego, CA 92198
www.ReferencePointPress.com

ALL RIGHTS RESERVED.
No part of this work covered by the copyright hereon may be reproduced or used in any form or by any means—graphic, electronic, or mechanical, including photocopying, recording, taping, web distribution, or information storage retrieval systems—without the written permission of the publisher.

LIBRARY OF CONGRESS CATALOGING-IN-PUBLICATION DATA

Names: Steffens, Bradley, 1955- author.
Title: Medical drones / by Bradley Steffens.
Description: San Diego, CA : ReferencePoint Press, Inc., 2020. | Series:
   World of drones | Includes bibliographical references and index.
Identifiers: LCCN 2019049334 (print) | LCCN 2019049335 (ebook) | ISBN
   9781682828311 (library binding) | ISBN 9781682828328 (ebook)
Subjects: LCSH: Medical technology. | Drone aircraft. | Medical
   care--Technological innovations. | Health services
   accessibility--Technological innovation.
Classification: LCC R855.3 .S74 2020 (print) | LCC R855.3 (ebook) | DDC
   610.285--dc23
LC record available at https://lccn.loc.gov/2019049334
LC ebook record available at https://lccn.loc.gov/2019049335

CONTENTS

Introduction   4
A New Era in Medical Care

Chapter 1   8
Transporting Organs for Transplants

Chapter 2   19
Delivering Medical Supplies

Chapter 3   31
Remote Testing and Care

Chapter 4   42
Medical Evacuations

Source Notes   53
For Further Research   57
Index   59
Picture Credits   63
About the Author   64

INTRODUCTION

A New Era in Medical Care

In May 2019 a seven-year-old boy at the New Tafo Government Hospital in eastern Ghana needed an immediate transfusion of O-negative blood. The hospital staff sent a frantic text message to a blood bank in the town of Omenako, an hour's drive away, requesting the blood. Less than fifteen minutes later, an unmanned aerial vehicle (UAV), or drone, appeared in the sky, cruising at an altitude of about 755 feet (230 m). As the sleek, white aircraft neared the hospital, it swooped down to an altitude of 33 feet (10 m) and opened a set of doors on its underside. A bright red box dropped from the cargo bay and parachuted to the ground. Inside was a package of O-negative blood, which the staff quickly administered to the boy. "If we hadn't gotten that, the child would have lost his life,"[1] says Kobena Wiredu, the hospital's medical superintendent.

> **altitude**
> The height of an object in relation to ground level

Medical Drone Networks

A drone is a UAV that is controlled either by an onboard computer or by a pilot on the ground, controlling the aircraft via radio signals. A drone can be a fixed-wing aircraft, similar to an airplane; it can have multiple, tiltable rotors, known as a rotorcraft; or it can have one or two fixed rotors, like a helicopter. The fixed-wing drone that delivered the lifesaving blood to the New Tafo hospital is owned and operated by Zipline International, an American company that is working with the Ghanaian government to improve the country's health care. Zipline opened its first Ghanaian distribution center in Omenako, 42 miles (68 km) north of Accra, the capital, in April 2019. The company plans to build three more centers. Eventually, Zipline will operate a fleet of thirty drones that will make six hundred flights each day, distributing blood, vaccines, and medication to two thousand Ghanaian hospitals and clinics that serve 20 million people. It will be the largest medical drone delivery network on the planet. But it is not the only one.

Zipline has been delivering blood by drone in Rwanda, more than 2,000 miles (3,219 km) southeast of Ghana, since 2016. Every day, Zipline drones deliver whole blood, plasma, and platelets to twenty-five Rwandan hospitals and clinics, making about four

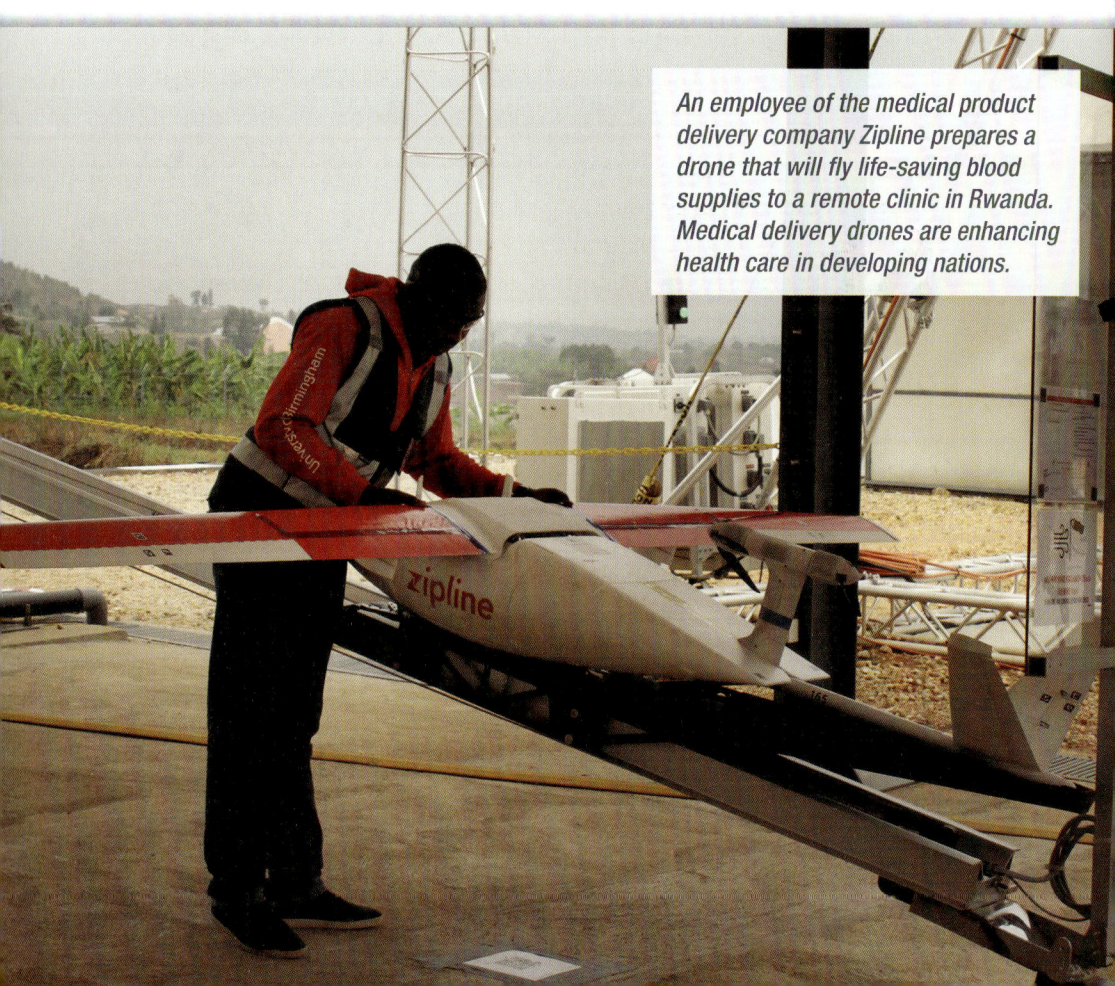

An employee of the medical product delivery company Zipline prepares a drone that will fly life-saving blood supplies to a remote clinic in Rwanda. Medical delivery drones are enhancing health care in developing nations.

thousand emergency deliveries a year. In Malawi, an African nation that has the world's ninth-highest rate of HIV/AIDS infection, drones are being used to transfer blood samples to and from hospitals to speed up HIV diagnoses in infants. In Papua New Guinea, an island nation in the Pacific, the international humanitarian organization Doctors Without Borders is using drones to transport samples from people suspected of having tuberculosis to hospitals for testing. In the Pacific island nation Vanuatu, the government has partnered with Australian drone maker Swoop Aero to deliver vaccines by drone to the country's eighty small islands.

Reaching the People in Need

Medical drones are part of a global strategy to bring quality health care to the developing nations of the world. Keller Rinaudo, Zipline's chief executive officer (CEO), says that today's advanced health care systems "really only serve the 'golden billion' people on the planet,"[2] referring mainly to the populations of Europe, North America, and Australia. Millions of people in rural Africa, Asia, and South America die each year from lack of access to vaccines, medications, blood transfusions, emergency care, and sophisticated diagnostics.

Drones may be able to change that. Guided by computers and Global Positioning System (GPS) data, drones can fly medical supplies to places that motor vehicles cannot go, in all kinds of weather, in the day or at night, dramatically reducing delivery time. "In many circumstances—say, a mother hemorrhaging after childbirth—a few seconds or minutes can mean the difference between life and death," says Robert Graboyes, a senior research fellow at George Mason University in Arlington, Virginia. "Across rugged terrain, traffic-clogged cities, icy roads or flooded regions, a drone may become the quickest and surest way to get medical goods to where they're needed."[3]

Improving Care in Advanced Nations

Drones have particular value in developing nations that lack medical infrastructure, but they may also have a role in improving health care in advanced countries. Matternet, a drone-delivery company based in Menlo Park, California, has teamed up with Swiss Post, the national postal service of Switzerland, to deliver medical supplies in three Swiss cities. Swiss Post says deliveries that used to take forty-five minutes by motor vehicle are now completed in a few minutes by drone.

> **infrastructure**
>
> The basic physical structures and facilities, such as roads, sewers, pipelines, and power plants, needed for the operation of a society

Drones are coming to the United States as well. Zipline is launching drone delivery programs to serve rural communities in Maryland, Nevada, and Washington. In March 2019 WakeMed Hospital in Raleigh, North Carolina, teamed up with Matternet and United Parcel Service (UPS) to use drones to speed up the delivery of medical samples across the hospital's sprawling 1-million-square-foot (92,903 sq. m) medical campus. In April 2019 researchers at the University of Maryland Medical Center conducted the first transplant of an organ delivered to a hospital by a drone.

While most medical drones are used outdoors, some researchers are working on small, indoor drones that could aid doctors, nurses, and patients. Some indoor drones are designed to carry medicine from the hospital pharmacy to drop-off points in the hospital, increasing the speed of delivery. Others are custom made to perform household tasks that might allow senior citizens to spend their final years at home, rather than in a nursing home. From delivering vaccines to remote islands to bringing elderly people their medications in their homes, drones are reshaping patient care around the world. Manohari Balasingam, a researcher at Kajang Hospital in Malaysia, believes that medical drones are opening a new era of medical care in much the same way as the first airplane flight at Kitty Hawk, North Carolina, opened a new era in transportation. "This," says Balasingam, "is a medical kitty hawk moment."[4]

CHAPTER 1

Transporting Organs for Transplants

Trina Glispy's medical ordeal began in 2011 with a simple injury that most people would recover from in a day or two at most. Then a thirty-six-year-old nursing assistant in Baltimore, Maryland, Glispy was kicked in the leg by a patient at work. While painful, a kicking injury usually results in nothing more than bruising. In Glispy's case, however, her leg swelled. After performing some tests, Glispy's doctors found that the swelling occurred because Glispy's kidneys were not removing excess water from her blood.

Healthy kidneys filter about 118 milliliters (about a half cup) of blood every minute. They remove waste and extra water from the bloodstream, making urine. Glispy's kidneys were not doing this, so doctors prescribed dialysis, a process in which a machine removes water and waste from the blood. Glispy began receiving dialysis treatments three times a week, with each session lasting four hours. Dialysis drained Glispy of energy, and she struggled to perform the physical labor required for the job that she loved.

Dialysis takes a heavy toll on the body. As a result, the average life expectancy for patients on dialysis is five to ten years, according to the National Kidney Foundation. At her age, with most of her life ahead of her, Glispy was the ideal candidate for a kidney transplant. In this procedure, a failing kidney is replaced by a kidney taken from either a living donor or a donor who has just died. The organ donor's blood type must match the blood type of the recipient. The donor's body size must match the recipient's as well, because a kidney that is too large or too small will not function properly in the recipient. With a successful transplant, the patient no longer needs dialysis. Kidney transplants often improve a patient's quality of life and can last for many years, although the patient might need another transplant in the future.

A kidney transplant is generally safe, but the wait to find a suitable kidney can be long. This is because the number of kidneys available for transplant is relatively small. According to the United Network for Organ Sharing (UNOS), which oversees the US transplant system, nearly 114,000 people are waiting for transplantable organs, including 93,000 who are waiting for kidneys. However, in 2018 only 36,500 organ transplants (of

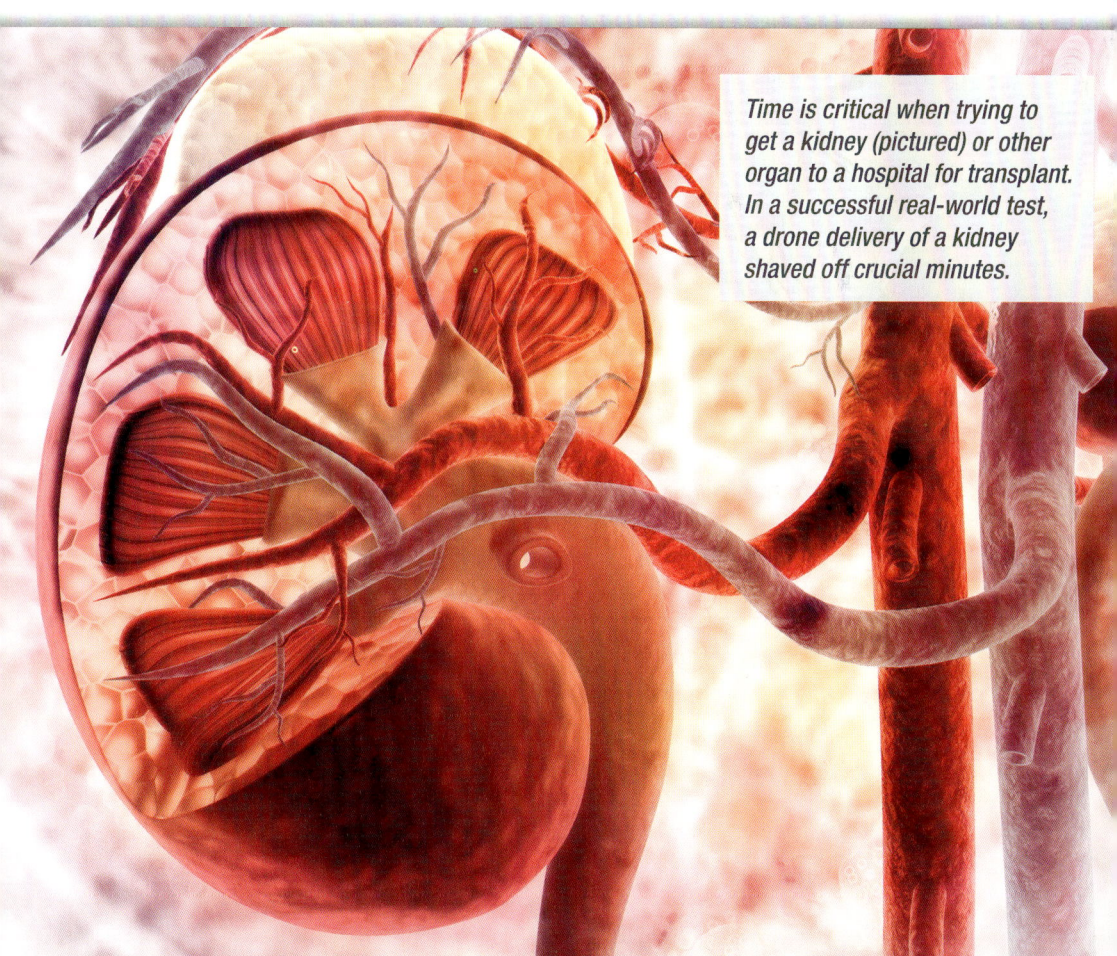

Time is critical when trying to get a kidney (pictured) or other organ to a hospital for transplant. In a successful real-world test, a drone delivery of a kidney shaved off crucial minutes.

all types) were performed. This was a historic high in the United States, but fell well short of the number of organs needed for transplants. The organ shortage means that people often must wait years for their transplant operations. The wait can be deadly. UNOS reports that in 2017 more than sixty-five hundred transplant candidates—an average of eighteen people a day—died while on the waiting list or within thirty days of leaving it for personal or medical reasons. Glispy had been waiting eight years for a transplant. She knew her time was running out. "I'm seeing a lot of people die and I'm like, 'It's taking so long, it might not happen for me either,'"[5] she says.

A Medical First

At 4:00 p.m. on April 18, 2019, Glispy got a call that a donor match had been found for her. She had to go to the hospital immediately to be prepared for surgery. The transplant team was assembled, and her doctors were ready to proceed. There was just one final step: the kidney had to be transported to the University of Maryland Medical Center, where the operation would take place.

An organ transport must be done quickly, because organs begin to deteriorate as soon as they're removed from the donor. The longer it takes to transport the organ, the lower the odds for a successful transplant. "We are very time sensitive," says Charlie Alexander, CEO of the Living Legacy Foundation of Maryland, the nonprofit organ procurement organization that obtained the kidney for Glispy. "We need to be able to work with helicopter services, charter flight services and ground transportation to make sure to get our teams to a donor case and make the gifted organ available to a recipient."[6]

In Glispy's case, moving the organ took just under ten minutes. This was due in part to the distance the organ had to travel—a mere 2.8 miles (4.5 km). It was also due to the mode of transportation used to deliver the organ. It was not driven to the hospital; it was flown by a drone, traveling 400 feet (122 m) above ground.

The Short Period of Organ Viability

An organ transplant involves removing a diseased organ from an ill patient and replacing it with a healthy organ from a deceased or living organ donor. (Most living donor transplants involve the surgical removal of one of a person's two kidneys, since the remaining kidney is able to perform the necessary functions.)

Preservation of the healthy organ is vital to the success of the transplant. To preserve the organ, the transplant team flushes it free of blood prior to its removal. The blood is replaced with an ice-cold preservation solution that contains electrolytes and nutrients. The organ is then placed in a sterile container and packaged in wet ice to keep it cool. The organ is then ready to be transported to the hospital where the transplant will take place.

Organs must be transported quickly because they begin to deteriorate immediately. Different organs can be preserved for different periods. Hearts and lungs must be transplanted within approximately four hours after being removed from the donor. Intestines can be preserved about eight hours, a pancreas can be preserved for about eight to twelve hours, livers can be preserved for twelve to eighteen hours, and kidneys can be preserved for twenty-four to forty-eight hours.

By the early hours of April 19, Glispy's transplant was complete. Five days later she was well enough to go home. "This whole thing is amazing," says Glispy. "Years ago, this was not something that you would think about."[7] Glispy told the *New York Times* that she was grateful for the lifesaving procedure. "I feel very fortunate, especially after watching so many people pass being on dialysis,"[8] she says.

The drone flight of the kidney Glispy received was not the result of a transportation emergency, but it was not a publicity stunt either. It was real-world test of a technology that researchers had been working on for months—one that could have far-reaching implications for the organ transplant field. "This is a major step towards reinventing the way that . . . organs are moved." says

Joseph Scalea, assistant professor of surgery at the University of Maryland School of Medicine and one of the surgeons who performed Glispy's transplant. "I think we can help a lot of people this way. It might take a long time, but it's a first step."[9]

A Custom Drone Design

The team led by Scalea took several precautions to ensure that the test would be successful. The drone, which researchers named the Human Organ Monitoring and Quality Assurance Apparatus for Long-Distance Travel (HOMAL), was custom built to hold the weight of the organ and monitoring devices. It had to follow Federal Aviation Administration (FAA) drone flying regulations and meet the medical, technical, and regulatory demands of carrying an unaccompanied deceased-donor organ for human transplant.

The drone was outfitted with backup propellers, motors, and batteries to complete the flight in case one or more of the primary components failed. It also was equipped with a parachute to bring it to earth without endangering the kidney in case all systems failed. "We always say 'we want to do no harm.' So, we have built a number of redundancies, because we want to do everything possible to protect the payload,"[10] says Anthony Pucciarella, director of operations at the Unmanned Aircraft Systems Test Site, part of the University of Maryland, College Park, where the drone was built.

The drone was controlled by a small onboard computer, but two pilots on the ground followed its progress using a wireless network. If a problem occurred, the pilots were ready to override the computer and guide the drone to its destina-

redundancy

The inclusion of extra components that are not strictly necessary for functioning, in case of failure in other components

payload

The part of a vehicle's load, especially an aircraft's, from which revenue is derived tion. As an added precaution, the Baltimore Police Department blocked ground traffic along the flight path while the aircraft flew overhead. As required by FAA regulations, the pilots maintained a visual line of sight on the drone throughout the flight.

To be sure they were ready for any possible problem, team members had tested the drone extensively before the lifesaving flight. The drone had logged more than seven hundred hours in forty-four test flights. Some test flights transported saline, blood, and other biological materials. In one of the tests, the drone carried a human kidney that could not be used for a transplant.

Keeping the Kidney Viable

The drone is only one part of a successful organ delivery. The container that holds the organ is equally important. The container had to keep the organ at a cool temperature, free of contamination, and at the proper air pressure. The HOMAL contained instruments to measure temperature, barometric pressure, altitude, vibration, and location via GPS during transportation. This information was sent directly to the smartphones of the transplant team so it could monitor the organ's status in real time. "When we started this project, I quickly realized there were a number of unmet needs in organ transport," says Scalea. "Even in the modern era, human organs are unmonitored during flight. I found this to be unacceptable. Real-time organ monitoring is mission-critical to this experience."[11]

Knowing the location of the organ and predicting its arrival time is also important. Scalea describes current organ transportation as "data-blind," meaning that doctors cannot see an organ's progress in transit.

barometric pressure

Another term for *atmospheric pressure*, the pressure exerted by the weight of the atmosphere, which at sea level is roughly 15 pounds (6.8 kg) per square inch

With the HOMAL, the surgeons receive updates the way a person might track a ride service on a cell phone. "We can monitor in real time," says Scalea. "It's like Uber for organs."[12]

While the University of Maryland's organ transport test was small, its success has large implications. "If we can prove this works, we can look at much greater distances of unmanned organ transport," says Alexander. "This would minimize the need for multiple pilots and flight time and address safety issues we have in our field."[13]

Transporting organs can be complicated. If a donor dies near the hospital where the transplant will be performed, the organ can be transported by ground vehicle. In some cases, such as those involving lungs, which can only remain viable for about four hours, the organ might be transported by a chartered helicopter to save time. If the donor dies in a distant, rural area, getting the organ to a hospital—usually a large hospital in a big city—is a

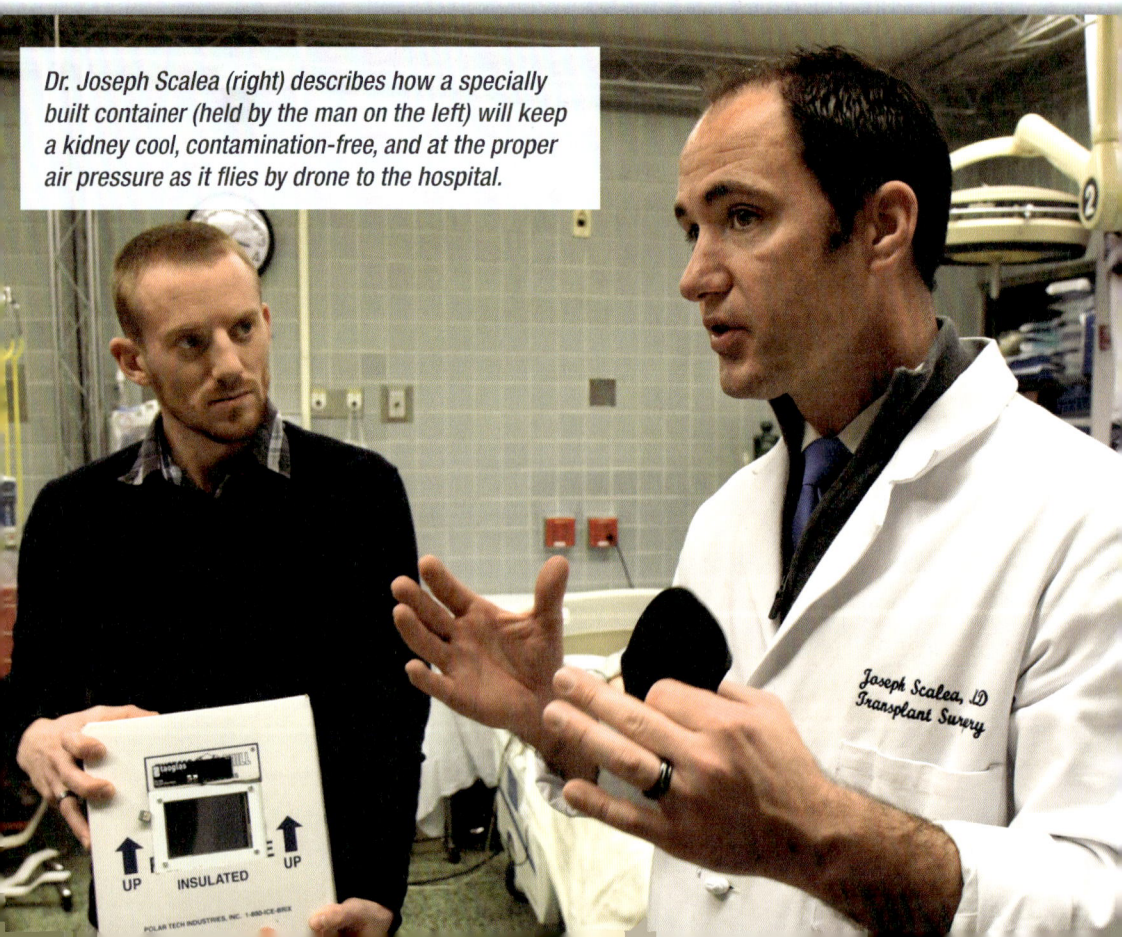

Dr. Joseph Scalea (right) describes how a specially built container (held by the man on the left) will keep a kidney cool, contamination-free, and at the proper air pressure as it flies by drone to the hospital.

major challenge. Some organs are sent in the cargo compartment of commercial airliners. Others travel via chartered jet. All of these modes of transportation have drawbacks. "Charters are too expensive, commercial aircraft is too slow and small aircraft at inconvenient hours are dangerous to transplant teams,"[14] says Scalea. He believes that long-range unmanned drone delivery could cut the time organs spend in transit by 70 percent.

Although organ transport usually goes smoothly, mistakes can be made. On December 9, 2018, a human heart was sent from Sacramento to Seattle in the cargo compartment of a Southwest Airlines flight. The heart was supposed to be offloaded in Seattle, but it remained on the plane when the aircraft left for Dallas, Texas. Airline employees realized the problem about ninety minutes into the flight to Dallas. The pilot made an announcement to passengers, turned the airliner around, and headed back to Seattle. Three hours had been lost in travel time, but the heart's valves were salvaged and later used in a transplant.

Scalea has seen firsthand what happens when organ transport takes too long. In one case, Scalea waited twenty-nine hours for a kidney from Alabama to reach his hospital in Baltimore. "Had I put that in at nine hours, the patient would probably have another several years of life,"[15] Scalea says. The case inspired Scalea to look into using drones to transplant organs. "Delivering an organ from a donor to a patient is a sacred duty with many moving parts," he says. "It is critical that we find ways of doing this better."[16]

Making More Transplants Possible

Speeding up the delivery of organs means that fewer will be wasted because it took too long to transport them to the hospital. As a result, more viable organs will be available for transplanting, and the number of patients who can receive the lifesaving operations will increase. Scalea estimates that rapid drone transport of "marginal" organs—organs that can only be used if there is no delay of any kind—could end up adding as many as twenty-five hundred kidneys a year to the donor pool. "There remains a woeful disparity between the number of recipients on the organ transplant waiting list and the total number of transplantable organs," says Scalea. "This new technology has the potential to help widen the donor organ pool and access to transplantation."[17]

Cost is another factor that affects how many people can receive transplants. Chartering private jets and helicopters is extremely expensive. Many patients cannot afford to transport the organs over great distances, so they must wait for them to become available locally. This puts the patients at a greater risk of dying before they receive a transplant. Unmanned drones can dramatically lower the cost of moving the donor organs, making the operation available to more patients.

Christopher Marsh, the director of the transplant program at Scripps Green Hospital in La Jolla, California, says that it is too soon to say for certain that unmanned drones will be a reliable way of delivering transplant organs over long distances. However, he believes drones hold promise for moving organs quickly from one hospital to another or from an airport to a hospital, avoiding big city traffic. "We're entering a new world," he says. "Things change, so we have to be open to that."[18]

Obstacles to Organ Delivery

Before organ delivery by drone can become commonplace, several obstacles need to be overcome. For one thing, drones must be able to fly farther and faster and carry bigger payloads. Scalea believes this is possible. "In the ideal world, I see drones moving 200 miles per hour and carrying payloads of 50–100 pounds, while still being able to land and take off vertically," Scalea says. "Those technologies are not yet available—although they are totally feasible."[19]

Even if drone technology can be upgraded to achieve such goals, the regulations governing their flights will have to change. One of the most important is the FAA regulation that requires drones to operate within the pilot's line of sight. Even if a pilot uses binoculars to watch the drone, the line-of-sight requirement limits the range of drone delivery to a few miles at most. To expand their range beyond the line of sight, drones need to be proved safe. "American skies can be crowded," says Robert Graboyes, a senior research fellow at George Mason University in Arlington, Virginia, "and the last thing the drone industry needs is a serious accident—a midair collision or a drone striking a building or person." Before the FAA will approve their long-range use, drones need to be equipped with reliable communications and collision avoidance systems. "The technology probably has to change in advance of wholesale regulatory reform,"[20] says Graboyes.

FAA Rules for Small Unmanned Aircraft

Small commercial drones, including medical delivery drones, must operate according to FAA rules that took effect in 2016. Some of the rules include the following:

- A person operating a small unmanned aerial system must be at least sixteen years old and hold a remote pilot airman certificate.
- Unmanned aircraft must weigh less than 55 pounds (25 kg).
- The maximum ground speed for unmanned aircraft is 100 miles per hour (87 knots).
- The maximum altitude for an unmanned aircraft is 400 feet (122 m) above ground level (AGL)—or, if higher than 400 feet AGL, it must remain within 400 feet of a structure.
- The minimum weather visibility allowed is 3 miles (4.8 km) from the control station.
- The unmanned aircraft must remain within the line of sight of the remote pilot in command.
- Small unmanned aircraft may not operate over any persons not directly participating in the operation.
- Unmanned aircraft are restricted to daylight-only operations, or twilight with appropriate anticollision lighting.
- Unmanned aircraft must yield the right of way to other aircraft.
- No person may act as a remote pilot in command for more than one unmanned aircraft operation at one time.
- Unmanned aircraft may not be operated from a moving aircraft.
- Unmanned aircraft may not be operated from a moving vehicle unless the operation is over a sparsely populated area.

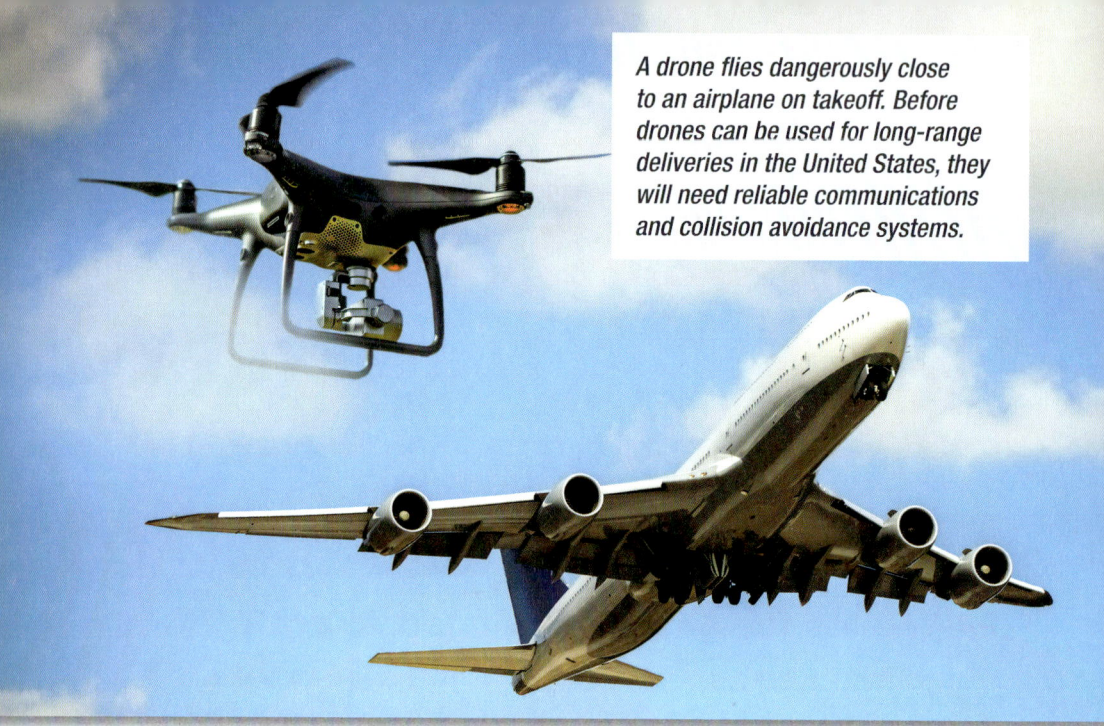

A drone flies dangerously close to an airplane on takeoff. Before drones can be used for long-range deliveries in the United States, they will need reliable communications and collision avoidance systems.

If drone transport is proved effective in the United States, it could open up the possibility of increased organ transplants not only in the developed world but also in less developed countries. Such countries may have hospitals where transplants can be performed but lack the infrastructure to enable donated organs to be delivered from outlying areas quickly enough for the organs to remain viable. In addition, drones could reduce the costs of moving organs in poor countries that lack the resources for medical aircraft and pilots. In other words, the Maryland drone experiment could help save lives around the world. "This history-making flight not only represents a breakthrough from a technological point of view, but provides an exemplary demonstration of how engineering expertise and ingenuity ultimately serve human needs—in this case, the need to improve the reliability and efficiency of organ delivery to hospitals conducting transplant surgery," says Darryll J. Pines, dean of the University of Maryland's A. James Clark School of Engineering. "As astonishing as this breakthrough is from a purely engineering point of view, there's a larger purpose at stake. It's ultimately not about the technology; it's about enhancing human life."[21]

CHAPTER 2

Delivering Medical Supplies

On December 18, 2018, Joy Nowai, a one-month-old baby in the island nation of Vanuatu, became the first person in history to be given a vaccine delivered by drone. The drone flew almost 25 miles (40 km) to deliver the vaccine to Cook's Bay, a remote area usually accessible only by foot or locally operated boats. A total of thirteen children and five pregnant women were vaccinated that day. "Today's first-of-a-kind vaccine delivery has enormous potential not only for Vanuatu, but also for the thousands of children who are missing out on vaccines across the world," said Henrietta H. Fore, executive director of the United Nations Children's Fund, an organization that provides food and health care to children around the world. "This is innovation at its best."[22]

Delivering vaccines, medications, and blood for emergency transfusions is currently the most common use for medical drones. In part this is because drones can reach places that land vehicles cannot—zipping over water, rough terrain, and dense jungle. It is also a matter of cost. Treating patients in place can be a lot less expensive than moving them to a hospital. Ryan Oksenhorn, a software developer with Zipline, says:

> It makes perfect sense to use this technology very cheaply and very quickly to travel long distances. Right now it costs $10,000 to emergency lift someone in a helicopter to go to the hospital if they need

blood. For [much] less money and less time you can deliver the blood with a drone. There's no need to send several humans in a helicopter. You can send the blood directly to the person who needs it.[23]

The First Large-Scale Medical Drone Network

Blood delivery is the first large-scale use of medical drones. Since 2016 a fleet of drones owned and operated by Zipline has been delivering whole blood, plasma, and platelets to hospitals and clinics in Rwanda, which has about the same area as the US state of Massachusetts. Due to the traffic and Rwanda's large number of unpaved roads, it can take up to five hours to deliver blood to a rural hospital by driving. That kind of wait can mean death to a patient who has lost a large amount of blood. "Patients frequently die because of lack of access to a basic medical product that exists in a central warehouse 75 kilometers away but can't make it out that final mile to the person who needs it,"[24] says Zipline CEO Keller Rinaudo. Zipline drones can reach almost any part of Rwanda in just forty-five minutes.

Zipline maintains 60 percent of Rwanda's blood products in two fulfillment centers, known as "nests." From there, the drones fan out across the country as needed. About half of the blood supply goes to treat mothers who are suffering from postpartum hemorrhaging, bleeding that sometimes occurs after giving birth. According to the Rwandan government, maternal mortality rates are declining thanks to the delivery of blood by drones.

Most Rwandan hospitals do not stock large supplies of blood, because the vital fluid has a short shelf life. It is also difficult to predict how much blood of each type will be needed over any given period. Holding large supplies of blood under ideal conditions and sending it to the hospitals by drone overcomes these problems. In its two years of operating at a national scale, Zipline's data show that it has helped Rwanda reduce its blood waste from about 7 percent to 0 percent. At an estimated cost of $80 to collect, test, and store a unit of blood, the reduction in wasted blood saves the Rwandan government more than $1 million per year.

Ground Operation

The Zipline nests receive shipments of blood by truck several times a week. When a shipment arrives, the workers quickly move the blood, plasma, and platelets into refrigerators. Hospitals can order the blood products by phone, text message, WhatsApp, or the company website. When an order is received, a staff member removes the blood products from the refrigerator, wraps them with padding, and places the bundle into a box with a wax-paper parachute attached. The box is loaded into the belly of the drone, known as a "Zip," and launched. The entire process takes about ten minutes.

Zipline's engineers believe the order fulfillment time can be much shorter. Israel Bimpe, Zipline's head of national implementation, says that changes in the procedure will eventually allow the company to fulfill orders in less than sixty seconds.

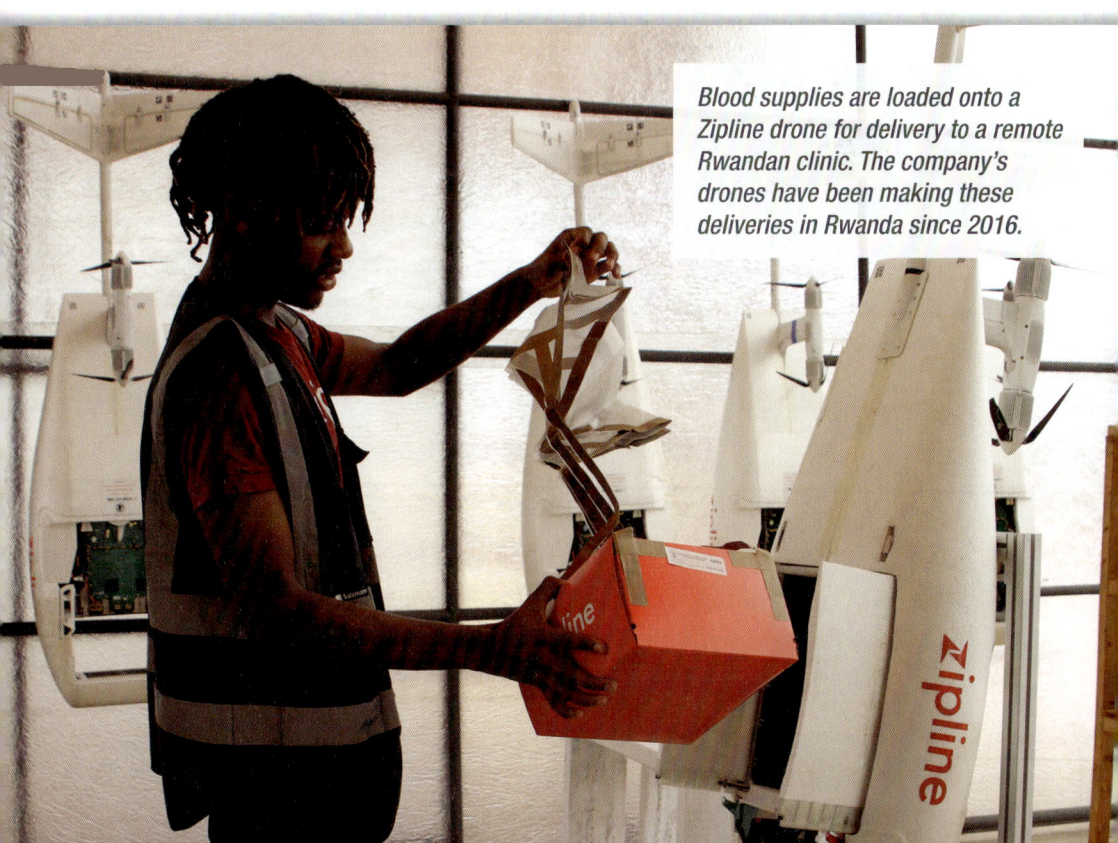

Blood supplies are loaded onto a Zipline drone for delivery to a remote Rwandan clinic. The company's drones have been making these deliveries in Rwanda since 2016.

"We just need to improve it a bit more," he says. "It's tweaking operational procedures and improving software to reduce that time to 1 minute. We receive an order and as soon as we finish packing, we just put it on the Zip and it's ready to go."[25]

Delivering blood products by drone makes sense in emergencies, when every moment counts. But drones cannot yet compete with motorbikes when it comes to moving large amounts of blood when there is ample time to do so. Right now, Zipline drones can carry a payload of only 2.9 pounds (1.3 kg), which amounts to two units of blood. Motorbikes can carry more than ten times that amount, about 33 pounds (15 kg), for routine deliveries. "Until you get to 6 or more likely 12 kg [for drones], it's not viable,"[26] says Jonathan Ledgard, the former director of African technology at the Swiss Federal Institute of Technology. The only

Launching a Drone

Drones with one propeller and fixed wings are ideal for long-distance medical deliveries because they fly faster and require less battery power. Technical experts Evan Ackerman and Michael Koziol describe the launch of a Zipline fixed-wing drone:

> A technician places the box and parachute in the belly of a drone behind a spring-loaded hatch, then snaps a modular battery pack into the drone's nose. Two people carry the drone to a 13-meter-long electric catapult powered by a bank of supercapacitors [devices that store and discharge electricity], then run through a preflight checklist with the aid of a smartphone app. Zipline confirms the drone's flight plan with the Rwanda Civil Aviation Authority and requests flight clearance. . . . Finally, with a satisfying zzzing, the catapult flings the drone skyward, accelerating it to 100 kilometers per hour in half a second.

Evan Ackerman and Michael Koziol, "In the Air with Zipline's Medical Delivery Drones," *IEEE Spectrum*, April 30, 2019. https://spectrum.ieee.org.

reason hospitals can afford Zipline blood products now is that the Rwandan government helps pay for the drone program. Ledgard says Zipline will have a hard time surviving if those payments end. "The price points they have to charge once the subsidies end are far, far, far too high for developing countries,"[27] Ledgard says.

The Next Generation of Zipline Drones

Zipline is already at work on a new generation of drones to better compete with land delivery. The new drones will have a lighter chassis and a more efficient battery. This will allow them to carry a payload of 3.9 pounds (1.75 kg), or three units of blood, an increase of 33 percent over the current drones. They will also be safer. They will be equipped with a transponder to sense and be located by other aircraft, a backup communication system that uses a satellite link rather than the cellular phone network, and sense-and-avoid equipment that will be able to automatically detect and avoid other aircraft. These will be important features as more drones and other aircraft take to the Rwandan skies.

transponder

A device for receiving a radio signal and automatically transmitting a response signal

The Rwandan government is confident that these improvements will make drone deliveries more efficient and economical. In 2019 the government awarded Zipline a three-year contract extension. New provisions call for Zipline to deliver not only blood products but also medicine and vaccines. The company will be adding new routes to its service, so it can deliver to small clinics as well as hospitals.

Zipline is partnering with a public-private global health partnership for the delivery of vaccines to remote areas of Rwanda. The group has been looking into using drones to deliver vaccines for several years, because the speed of the delivery can mean the difference between life and death. For example, a child who is bitten by a rabid animal must receive the rabies vaccine as quickly as possible. Drones can deliver the vaccine in a fraction of the time it takes a motor vehicle. "The global health community is looking for new ways to deliver vaccines, increase coverage and protect children against various diseases," says the group's spokesperson Frédérique Tissandier. "With all the mountains in Rwanda it's hard to get to remote villages. Some places can only be reached by boat. We're using this partnership to save kids' lives and protect them from vaccine-preventable disease."[28]

Medical Delivery in Ghana

Rwanda is not the only country using drones to improve its health care. At the end of 2018, the government of Ghana approved a four-year contract with Zipline to deliver medical supplies by drone. The drones will carry not only blood products, but also vaccines, antivenom, birth control pills, and condoms.

According to the World Health Organization, there were about 270 cases of malaria per 1,000 people in Ghana in 2017. The malaria rate in rural areas, where 45 percent of Ghanaians live, is even higher than the national average. Malaria is preventable and curable, but getting supplies such as medications and blood to rural Ghanaians is difficult. Most of Ghana's remote communities are connected to cities and towns by dirt roads. In the rainy season, many of these roads are flooded, and some are impassable. But drones, which can fly in by day or night and in all kinds of weather, can reach such communities easily. "During the rainy season, we have a lot more malaria cases. We tend to use a lot of blood," says George Appiah Boadu, a medical laboratory scientist at the New Tafo Government Hospital. "Now we are not going to have to rely on the roads. It's a huge relief to us and our patients."[29]

Not everyone supports Ghana's drone program. Critics say that the money the government is spending on drones would be better spent on health infrastructure. The Ghana Medical Association, a network of health professionals, believes staffing is a more critical need than drones. It says that some of the hospitals receiving drone deliveries do not have enough trained staff to administer the medical supplies once they arrive. "The use of drones without the necessary improvement in the human resource capacity will not [be of benefit to] the country,"[30] says the Ghana Medical Association in a statement.

Ghanaian president Nana Akufo-Addo admits that the country lacks critical medical infrastructure. For example, it now has only fifty-five ambulances serving the entire country. But he defends the use of drones as a way to save lives now. "No one in Ghana should die because they can't access the medicine they need in an emergency," says Akufo-Addo. "That's why Ghana is launching the world's largest drone delivery service . . . a major step towards giving everyone in this country universal access to lifesaving medicine."[31]

Treating Heart Attacks

Currently, drones are mainly used to carry lightweight medical payloads, including blood, vaccines, snakebite antivenom, and other medications. Some medical drone experts are building drones to carry heavier payloads. Mark Head, foreign crisis coordinator for RAM, a nonprofit organization that provides medical care to remote areas, is especially interested in using drones to deliver automated external defibrillators (AEDs) to remote areas.

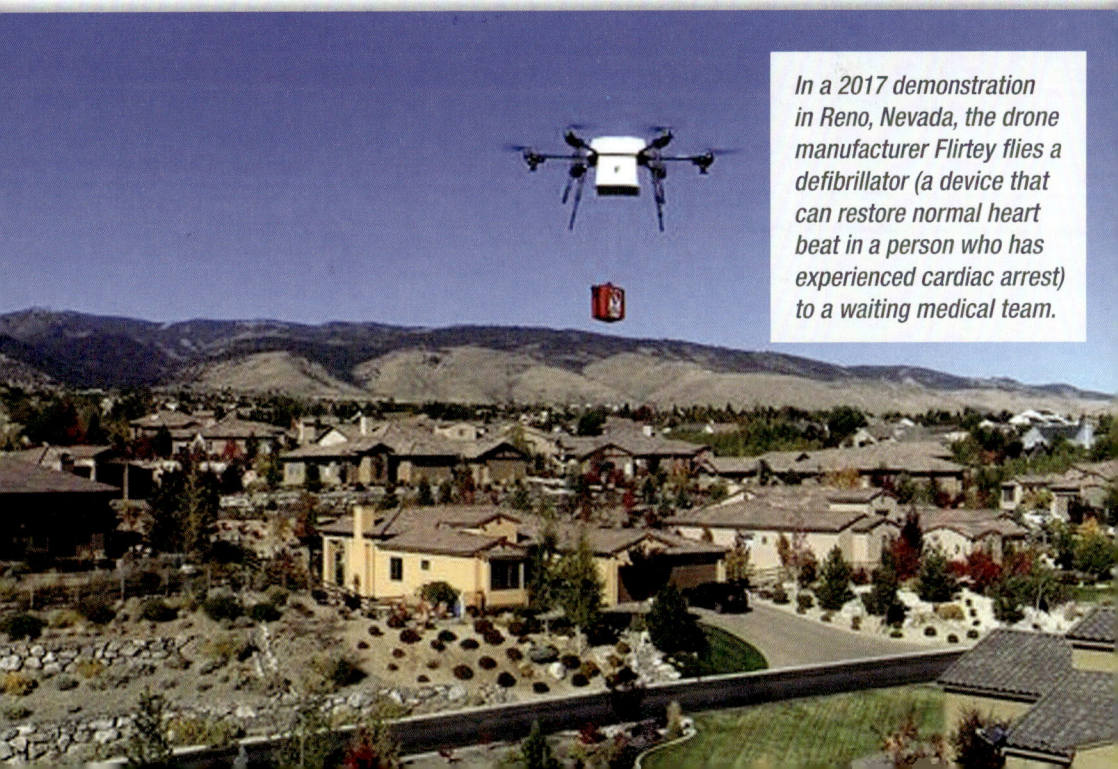

In a 2017 demonstration in Reno, Nevada, the drone manufacturer Flirtey flies a defibrillator (a device that can restore normal heart beat in a person who has experienced cardiac arrest) to a waiting medical team.

AEDs are portable devices that deliver an electric shock through the chest to the heart to normalize an irregular heartbeat after a heart attack. "If you can get a drone to a downed person having a heart attack quicker than an ambulance, you can save lives," Head says. "The thing about a defibrillator is it doesn't matter how you use it as long as you can get to the patient quickly. It's the time after the event that's critical."[32]

Cardiac arrest, an abrupt loss of heart function, is the third-leading natural cause of death in the United States behind cancer and other heart disease, according to the Health and Medicine Division (HMD) of the National Academies of Sciences, Engineering, and Medicine. Treating cardiac arrest quickly is vital. According to the HMD, for every minute that passes until a cardiac arrest victim receives defibrillation, his or her odds of survival decrease by about 10 percent. Deploying AEDs via drones can increase the average survival rate for cardiac arrests

Capturing a Drone

Drones equipped with vertical rotors can descend straight down and land softly, but fixed-wing drones cannot do this. A fixed wing drone—the type used for delivering medical supplies—could land on a runway like an airplane, but landing gear is heavy and limits how much cargo a drone can carry. Instead of landing, fixed-wing drones are snatched out of the air as they fly over a landing area.

To capture its fixed-wing drones, Zipline uses a system nicknamed Tall Bob. It consists of two 33-foot-high (10 m) towers, each with a rotating arm attached to it. A cable is strung between the two arms. Each drone has a small metal hook attached to the underside of its tail, similar to the tail hook on military jets that land on aircraft carriers. As the drone flies between the towers, Tall Bob's arms swing up, raising the cable until it snags on the drone's tail hook. The cable pulls the drone to a stop, and the rotating arms allow it to drop onto a large cushion. The entire process takes less than a second. The workers unhook the drone and reset the arms so Tall Bob is ready to capture the next drone.

that occur outside a hospital setting from just 10 percent to approximately 47 percent.

To increase the cardiac arrest survival rate, RAM has been working with Dennis Strege, owner of drone maker MasterFlight, to build a bigger, more powerful drone that is capable of carrying an AED. Strege is starting with a drone originally built to inspect power lines. The modified craft will be able to carry a 55-pound (25 kg) payload up to 150 nautical miles (278 km) in all kinds of weather, including conditions that would keep light airplanes and helicopters grounded.

Australian drone manufacturer Flirtey has also designed a drone to ferry defibrillators to places they are needed. On March 8, 2019, Flirtey announced that the FAA will allow the company to conduct drone delivery flights beyond visual line of sight for an experimental program in Reno, Nevada. Unlike many drones, the ones approved by the FAA will not be guided by automated systems. Instead, a pilot must control the flight from a remote location on the ground, using onboard cameras and GPS tracking to navigate safely to the destination.

The Reno pilot program was approved in part because of its lifesaving potential. According to Reno's historical data, just one AED delivery drone could save a life every two weeks in the city. Deployed nationwide, AED drones have the potential to save more than 100,000 lives per year and more than 1 million lives over each decade to come. "Public safety is our top priority, and the use of drones to provide life-saving AED technology to cardiac patients will save lives across our community,"[33] says Reno mayor Hillary Schieve.

Pilot Programs in the United States

One of the reasons that many drone programs have been launched in developing countries is that the governments have been flexible when it comes to regulating the unmanned craft. Advanced countries, with more air traffic to worry about, have been slower to approve their use. In the United States, the FAA is beginning to allow pilot programs like the one in Reno to see whether drones can be safely integrated into the nation's busy airspace.

In July 2015 Flirtey, the Mid-Atlantic Aviation Partnership at Virginia Tech, and the National Aeronautics and Space Administration's (NASA) Langley Research Center in Hampton, Virginia, held an event called Let's Fly Wisely to demonstrate the potential of delivering medical supplies by drone. NASA flew a fixed-wing drone carrying medical supplies from Langley to Lonesome Pine Airport, a one-runway airport in the small town of Wise, Virginia, over 400 miles (644 km) away. There the medical cargo was transferred in smaller packages and flown by drones to the Wise County Fairgrounds, where two local health care organizations were holding a free medical clinic for about fifteen hundred people. It was the first time a drone delivered medical supplies and pharmaceuticals in the United States. "In that part of Virginia (where Let's Fly Wisely took place), a large number of underserviced people can't get out of the house during the winter, particularly during inclement weather, but are in desperate need of blood pressure medicine or whatever medicine it is," says Stan Brock, founder and president of RAM, a nonprofit organization that provides medical care to remote areas. "A drone could take that medicine to them where a vehicle wouldn't be able to do so."[34]

airspace

The air available for aircraft to fly in, especially the part subject to the jurisdiction of a particular country

Medical experts believe that technology will enable outpatient care and home-based care that is currently delivered only in a hospital. Drones could contribute to this capability and make it safer. For example, a health care provider who visits a home patient might order medications, antibiotics, or other treatment, which could be delivered by drone while the provider is there to administer them. A drone could possibly even deliver a meal to a patient who cannot prepare his or her own meals.

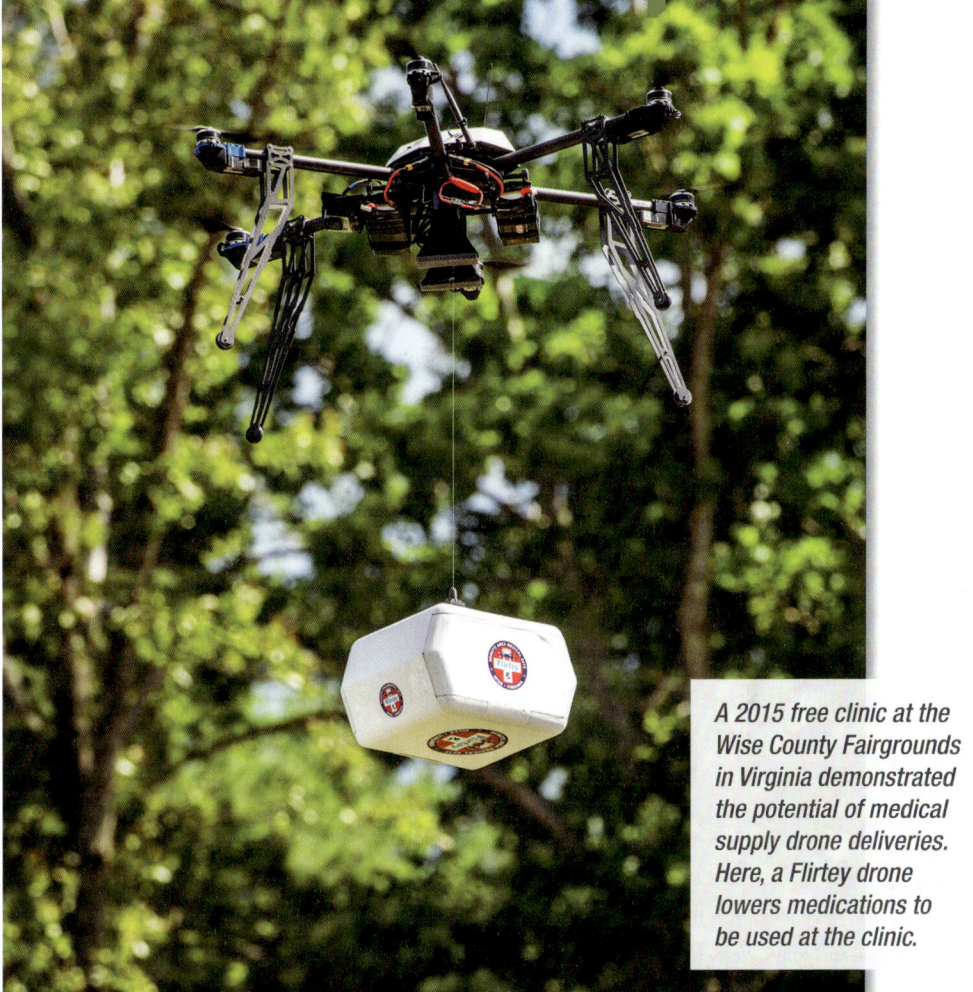

A 2015 free clinic at the Wise County Fairgrounds in Virginia demonstrated the potential of medical supply drone deliveries. Here, a Flirtey drone lowers medications to be used at the clinic.

Indoor Drone Deliveries

Most drone deliveries take place outdoors, with drones flying over miles of rough terrain, but some health care experts see drones performing important tasks indoors, within hospitals. Rather than having a hospital staffer, sometimes known as a pharmacy porter, load up a cart with patient medications and then deliver them on foot throughout the hospital—a slow process—some experts foresee using drones to deliver the drugs. In this scenario, the pharmacy porter would never leave the pharmacy. Instead, he or she would affix the medications to small indoor drones. The drones would carry the medications directly to the nurses requesting them, eliminating the wait for delivery by cart. Since fewer people would handle the drugs in transit, the chances for error would be decreased. "Nurses and pharmacists can work more efficiently as supplies can be summoned to the bedside instead of the time consuming task of gathering necessary items,"[35] says Jeremy Tucker, chair of the Emergency Department and Physician Champion for Patient Safety at MedStar St. Mary's Hospital in Leonardtown, Maryland.

pneumatic tubes

Systems that propel cylindrical containers through networks of tubes by compressed air or by creating a partial vacuum

Some hospitals use pneumatic tubes to send drugs from the pharmacy to nursing stations. The delivery to the patient's room must then be made by a nurse. "As the technology continues to advance, a small drone can be scheduled to deliver medicine at 3 in the afternoon to room X," says Will Stavanja, founder of consulting company Wilstair. "As long as each of the waypoints are programmed for the drone's trajectory, the drone can complete operations a pneumatic tube can't."[36] Drone delivery could be particularly helpful to hospitals that need to add additional space. Expanding a pneumatic tube system is expensive compared to the cost of using a fleet of small indoor drones.

Indoors or out, medical treatment is always a race against time. Unimpeded by bad roads, heavy traffic, rivers, oceans, and other phenomena that slow traditional delivery of medical supplies, drones have the ability to win that race against time. In doing so, medical drones will save countless lives.

CHAPTER 3

Remote Testing and Care

Every day, drones deliver lifesaving medical supplies—blood, plasma, antivenom, rabies vaccines, and more—to patients around the world. But before a treatment can be administered, the health care professional must know what a patient is suffering from and how advanced the condition is. For some conditions, such as a severe injury, the doctor can simply look at the patient and determine what treatment is needed. For other conditions, such as infectious illness, a doctor might check the patient's temperature, blood pressure, heart rate, or other things. But for many medical conditions, physicians must run tests. To do so, they might collect samples of a patient's blood, urine, stool, saliva, or even hair. As with treatment, delivering the samples to a testing laboratory and receiving the results is often a race against time. Drones are being used to win this race as well.

Testing Drone Delivery in North Carolina

In March 2019 WakeMed Hospital in Raleigh, North Carolina, teamed up with UPS and drone maker Matternet to use drones to speed up the delivery of medical samples to the hospital's laboratory. It is the first revenue-producing drone flight program approved by the FAA. Eight times a day, the drones carry small coolers of medical samples to a laboratory three-quarters of a mile away. A courier vehicle takes ten to twenty minutes for the driver to receive the samples, walk to the vehicle, drive to the laboratory, park, and go inside to deliver the sample. A drone completes the delivery in four minutes. "We are interested in speed and reliability," says Stuart Ginn, a physician and the driving force behind the program. "We're talking about shaving off 30 minutes to three hours easily, from our lab, end-to-end lab time."[37] Faster delivery of samples means faster test results and faster answers for doctors and patients.

The WakeMed program is a three-year pilot program designed to test whether medical drones can be safely integrated into the Raleigh airspace. If the program succeeds, Ginn would like to see it expanded so that samples could be flown between hospitals located miles apart. Eventually, samples gathered in rural areas could be flown by drone to large hospitals for testing. "So maybe the patient doesn't even have to come here. And maybe they can be cared for at that smaller facility,"[38] Ginn says.

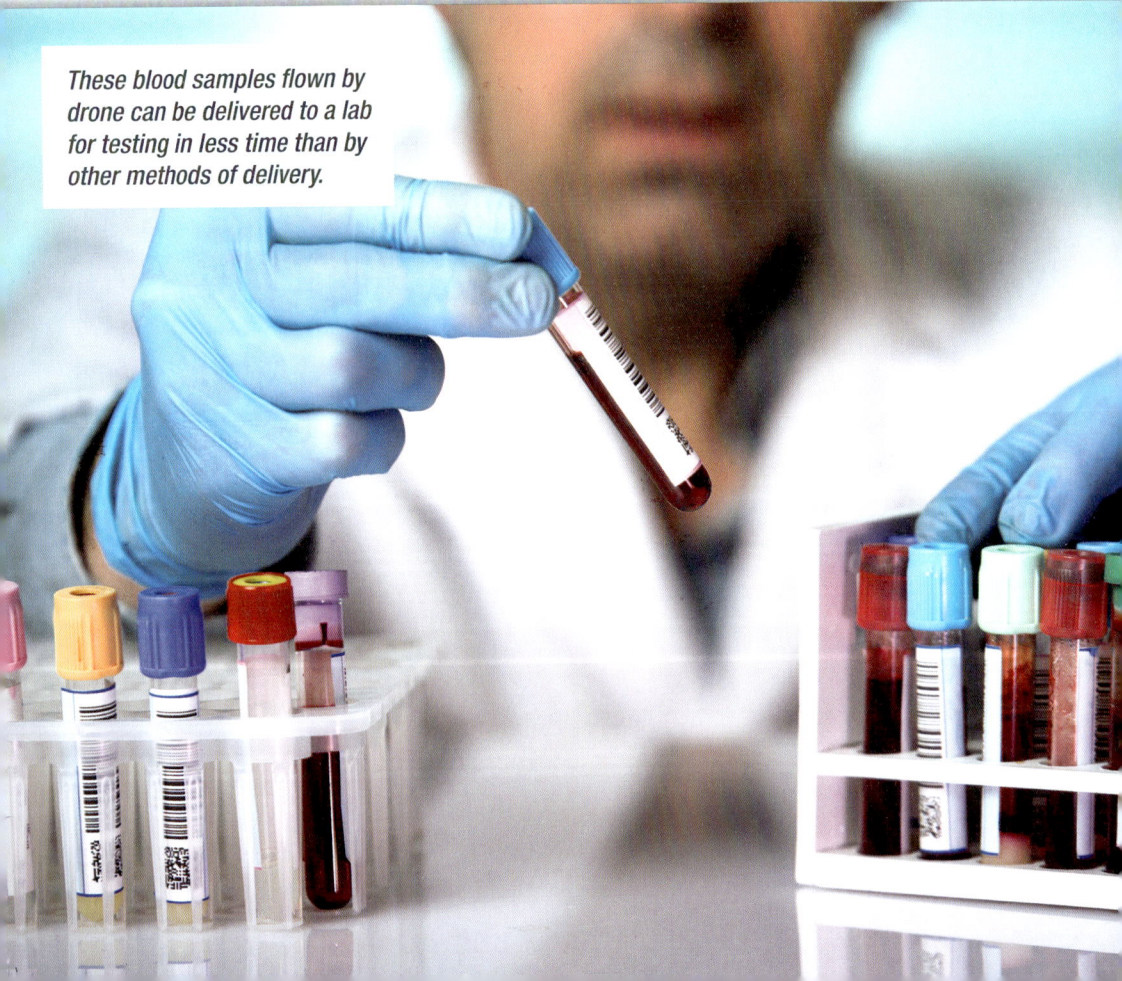

These blood samples flown by drone can be delivered to a lab for testing in less time than by other methods of delivery.

A Need for Speed

Medical testing has become even more important in this century, since the number of people dying from noncommunicable diseases such as cancer, heart disease, and diabetes has surpassed the number of people dying from infectious diseases such as HIV/AIDS or tuberculosis for the first time in history. According to the World Health Organization, noncommunicable diseases kill 38 million people worldwide each year. Since noncommunicable diseases develop over a person's lifetime, people need to be tested for them periodically. If discovered early, these diseases often can be treated successfully. Early discovery requires biological samples to be taken from a patient and tested in a lab. Drones can assist with this by carrying samples from remote areas to testing facilities quickly. "Speed is everything," says Timothy Amukele, a pathologist at Johns Hopkins University. "If it sits there for a long time, at some point the specimen starts deteriorating. It's not so useful anymore."[39]

Even in the United States, increasing the speed, quality, and number of medical tests can save lives. Zipline's Keller Rinaudo believes that by bringing medical testing to remote areas, drones can play a significant role in improving health outcomes. "When you look at rural or isolated communities, particularly Native American populations, populations that live on islands, you have serious health outcome inequalities," says Rinaudo. "There's a linear relationship between how far away you live from a city and your expected lifespan. So our hope is that this type of technology can solve those kinds of inequalities."[40]

The feasibility of using drones to transport samples to laboratories from remote islands was tested in 2016 by Johns Hopkins University School of Medicine and the nonprofit Field Innovation Team. The researchers used Flirtey drones to fly simulated samples from an onshore medical camp at Cape May, New Jersey, to a test facility on a vessel off the New Jersey coast. The drones then flew medical supplies back to the camp, where they could be used for treatment. The test suggests that floating labs equipped with drones could bring medical care to remote islands, such as the Aleutian Islands in Alaska.

Medical Lockbox

Drone delivery of medications and medical supplies is essential to the vision of allowing more older people to live at home, rather than in nursing homes. However, such deliveries must be secure. Drugs and medical supplies are expensive, and leaving them on an elderly person's porch can be an open invitation to thieves. To make medical deliveries more secure, Brandon Pargoe of Glen Allen, Florida, invented AirBox, a solar-powered lockbox designed to work with delivery drones.

The AirBox uses cell phone technology to have a delivery drone sent to its location using GPS coordinates. As the delivery drone approaches, the doors of the lockbox open automatically. The drone drops its cargo into the open box. When the package lands inside the AirBox, it closes and locks its doors, and the drone flies away. The lockbox then sends a delivery notification to the recipient's cell phone. The message includes an encrypted code, which the recipient can use to open the lockbox and retrieve the package.

The lockbox is an important step in making home care a reality. "[For] home bound patients, there won't be the constant need of family members to take them to the pharmacy and get them to places that they need," explains Pargoe.

Quoted in Heather Sullivan, "Local Invention to Help Deliver Medicines in Africa & Caribbean," NBC 12, November 16, 2018. www.nbc12.com.

Testing the Effects of Drone Flight on Samples

The Core Laboratory at Johns Hopkins Hospital in Baltimore has also tested the feasibility of using drones to transport biological samples within urban areas, where street traffic can slow delivery by traditional means. When a patient has blood drawn or provides a urine sample at a doctor's office, the tests of the sample are rarely done at that location. Some clinics can perform some tests on the premises, but not all. In those cases samples must be sent to more sophisticated labs.

In the Core Laboratory test, the researchers took six blood samples from fifty-six volunteers at Johns Hopkins Hospital. Half of the samples from each patient were taken directly to the hospital's lab for immediate analysis. The other samples were packed in foam and surrounded by a sponge that would fully absorb the blood in case of accident. The samples were then loaded on a drone and flown around for various periods of time, from six to thirty-eight minutes.

Researchers were interested in finding whether changes in air pressure, vibrations caused by the drone's motors, or the jostling at takeoff and landing would affect the samples. The researchers compared the flown samples to the samples sent directly to the laboratory to see whether the samples had deteriorated. They had not. Amukele, who led the experiment, was pleased with the outcome. He foresees a day when moving samples by drone will be commonplace. "A drone is a transport mechanism," says Amukele. "I think in 5–10 years it will be just like having a motorcycle, where it doesn't matter what you put on it, as long as you package it safely."[41]

Drones and Telemedicine

Laboratory tests are not required for every diagnosis, of course. Doctors diagnose patients all the time just by meeting with them and examining them. Technology like computerized video chats and medical cell phone applications are now allowing doctors to diagnose patients from a distance. This process is known as telemedicine. Italo Subbarao, senior associate dean at William Carey University College of Osteopathic Medicine in Hattiesburg, Mississippi, believes that telemedicine can be improved by using drones.

Subbarao is developing drones with video cameras, diagnostic equipment, and emergency medical supplies, including medications, bandages, gauze, clotting sponges,

telemedicine

The remote delivery of health care services, such as health assessments or consultations, over the telecommunications infrastructure

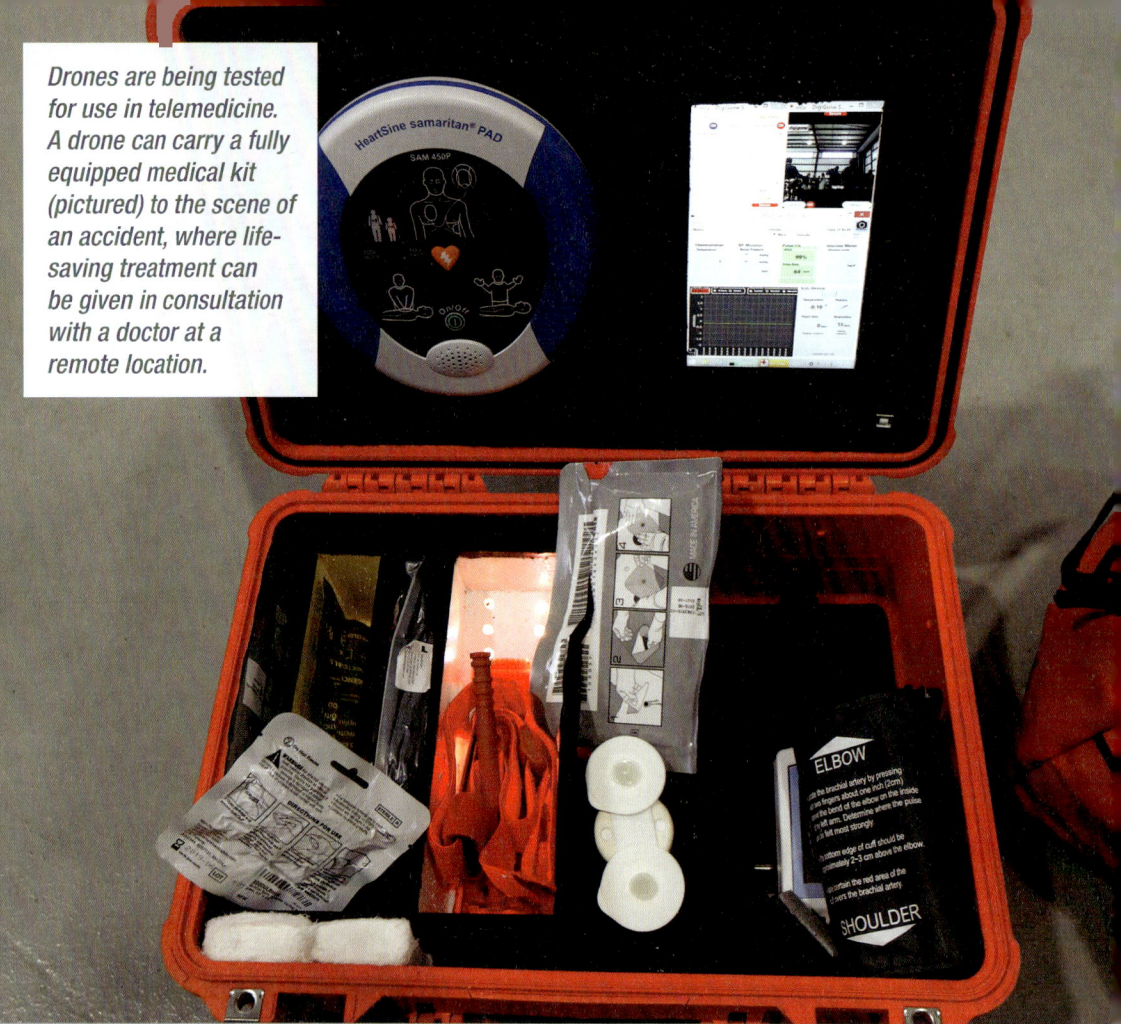

Drones are being tested for use in telemedicine. A drone can carry a fully equipped medical kit (pictured) to the scene of an accident, where life-saving treatment can be given in consultation with a doctor at a remote location.

scissors, and tourniquets. The drones would fly to emergency situations, such as an automobile accident, after being summoned by a 911 call. Not only would the drone bring medical supplies, but a doctor would be present via a two-way video chat to provide an immediate diagnosis. "A telemedical drone is the bridge that can deliver life-saving treatment directly to the victims, giving remote physicians eyes, ears, and voice to instruct anyone on site,"[42] says Subbarao.

Using the high-powered camera in Google Glass, the physician would see what a wound looks like and determine the nature of the injury. The doctor would then communicate with people at the accident site, telling willing bystanders what they can do to help and even guiding them through the appropriate treatments. "Drones have been used for awhile to get eyes on disaster scenes fast, so we thought, 'Why not integrate medical intervention as well?'" Subbarao says. "Why can't we use drones to deliver telemedical packages? Not just bandages and blood, or even a defibrillator, but on-site medical expertise, to give people on the scene a real medical intervention capability?"[43]

Subbarao and his team have created two different telemedical packages. One is designed to provide emergency care to a small number of severely injured victims. The other is intended to help up to one hundred people with moderate to minor injuries, as might be seen in a mass casualty event such as a train accident, an explosion, or an earthquake. "Immediate communications with the victims and reaching them rapidly with aid are both critical to improve outcomes,"[44] says Subbarao.

The drones used in the telemedical program are being built at nearby Hinds Community College in collaboration with Subbarao and his team of researchers. Each disaster drone is 3 feet (0.91 m) tall and 6 feet (1.8 m) in diameter. Powered by eight engines, the drones are designed to fly in all kinds of weather. The drones are equipped with GPS navigation so they can fly directly to the scene of the accident using the GPS coordinates of the cell phone that was used to call emergency services. The drones carry a variety of sensors, including infrared devices, to help locate victims in the dark. The drones have the ability to land in places that emergency medical service ground vehicles cannot get to or take too long to reach.

As with other drones being deployed in the United States, the telemedical drones are limited by FAA regulations that restrict privately owned drones to a maximum weight of 55 pounds (25 kg) and an altitude ceiling of 400 feet (122 m) above the ground or

infrared

A type of electromagnetic radiation, sometimes called infrared light, with longer wavelengths than those of visible light and therefore generally invisible to the human eye

Inspired by *Cinderella*

Naira Hovakimyan, a professor in mechanical science and engineering at the University of Illinois at Urbana-Champaign, has led a team of researchers to develop small drones, about the size of a person's hand, to fly indoors and perform tasks for the elderly. The goal is to provide enough assistance to allow the elderly to continue living in their homes, rather than having to move into a nursing home. Hovakimyan says that the inspiration for her flying robots came from the most unlikely of places: the animated Walt Disney movie *Cinderella*. Hovakimyan explains, "If you remember, Cinderella was being helped by mice and birds. So, we thought that if Cinderella could be helped by mice and birds, then ground robots and drones can help the elderly in their daily lives and secure independent aging at residences for longer periods."

Quoted in David Robertson, "Bibbidi Bobbidi Bots: ASPIRE to Improve Lives of Senior Citizens," Coordinated Science Laboratory, August 13, 2015. https://csl.illinois.edu.

buildings. The FAA also requires that the pilot be able to maintain visual contact with the drone throughout its flight. The line-of-sight requirement is the biggest problem. "We need to get beyond line-of-sight to using GPS guidance to direct the drones to the coordinates of the emergency call," says Dennis Lott, director of Hinds Community College's UAV program. He believes that when drones are equipped with collision avoidance systems, the FAA will permit their use beyond the sight line. "In any case, we think it's just a matter of time before drone technology is universally adopted for emergency and disaster response,"[45] Lott says.

Providing In-Home Care with Drones

Once diagnostic drones have proved themselves in emergency situations, they might become commonplace in other kinds of telemedicine. This could include, for example, the growing US senior population, age sixty-five and older, which is estimated to reach 71 million by 2030. A team of researchers at the University of Illinois at Urbana-Champaign, led by Naira Hovakimyan, a professor in mechanical science and engineering, is designing indoor drones to provide care to the elderly. The drones are equipped with a robotic arm that can be used to give the patient medication, bring a glass of water, pick up items from the floor, and even sort laundry. The idea is to provide a way for seniors to spend their final years at home, rather than in a nursing home. "The idea is that if we get technologically equipped houses, people will most likely enjoy their independent life in their home as opposed to going to a nursing home, where things will be overstuffed and understaffed,"[46] says Hovakimyan.

The biggest and most important challenge of providing in-home care with drones is patient safety. Unlike hospitals, which have wide hallways and high ceilings that can accommodate indoor drones, most homes have limited aerial space. To map out acceptable flight paths within homes, the University of Illinois team is first testing the concept with virtual reality headsets that create a three-dimensional simulation of a situation. The researchers show people a virtual reality simulation with in-home drones and use head-tracking software and body sensors to monitor how people react to the drones. "We're immersing people in virtual reality where these drones are flying around them," Hovakimyan explains. "Depending on people's reaction, including heart rate and head tilt, we can revise the drone design to make sure it's safe for people."[47]

For the program to work, the patients must feel comfortable interacting with the robotic drone. To this end, the University of Illinois team is studying how drones' appearance and behavior influence humans' perception of them. "If I talk today to the elderly about bringing drones into their houses to fly to help them, they will

head-tracking software

Technology that uses electronic sensors to determine how the user's head is moving during a virtual reality session

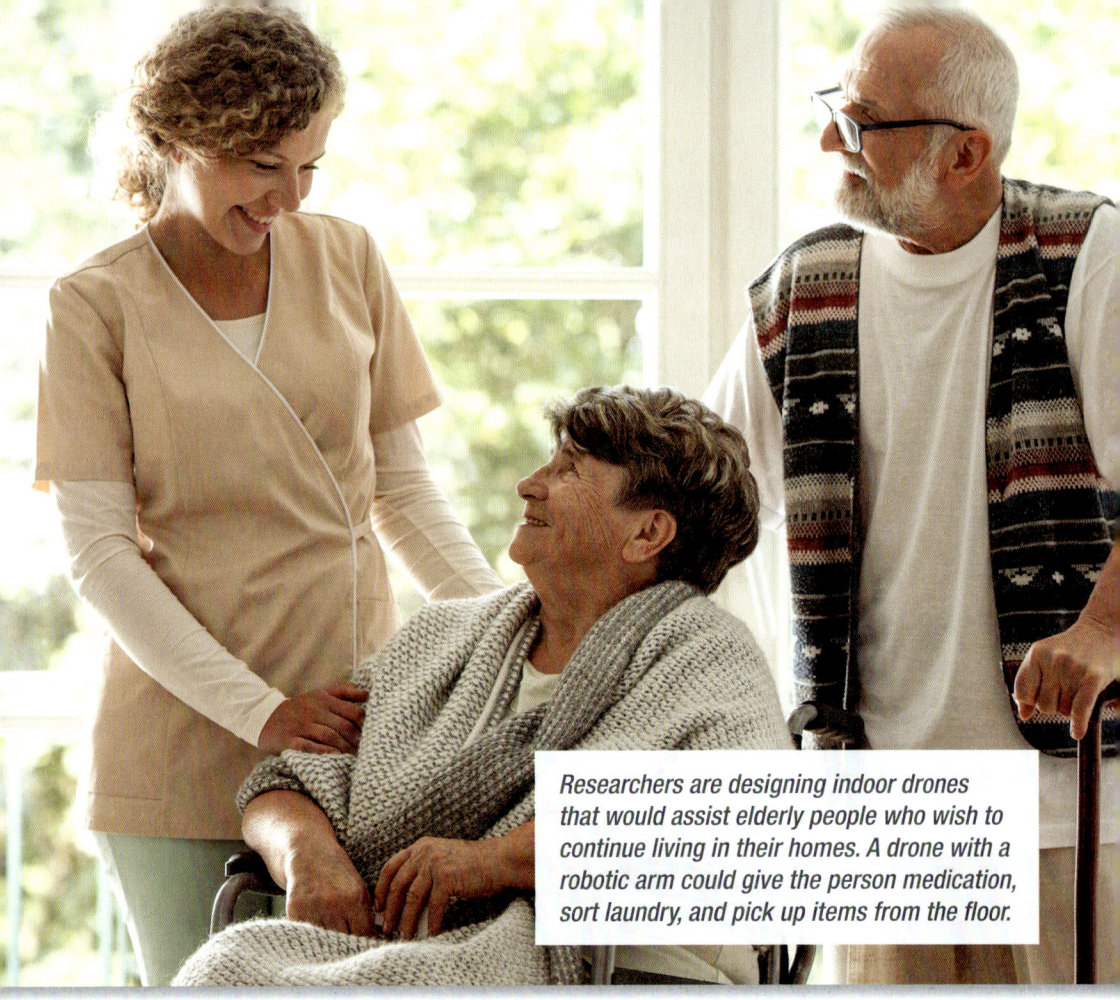

Researchers are designing indoor drones that would assist elderly people who wish to continue living in their homes. A drone with a robotic arm could give the person medication, sort laundry, and pick up items from the floor.

be scared of it," says Hovakimyan. "We must have a soft, nice flying system."[48] Appropriately, the title of Hovakimyan's in-home drone program is NICER, for Non-Intrusive Cooperative Empathetic Robots. "We want our robots to be non-intrusive and to blend in with the decor of the home," says Hovakimyan. "In order to achieve this goal, we need to understand the psychological aspects that lie behind Man-Robot interaction."[49]

Finding a Place for Drones in Health Care

From couriers who deliver medical samples to nurses who deliver in-home care, medical staffing is one of the most expensive elements of health care. To control costs, health care organizations will likely use technology to deliver services, and drones will be part of that process. "Drones are going to decrease the reliance on human beings that provide care and decrease the cost of assisting people,"[50] says Jeremy Tucker.

Specially modified drones have proved themselves capable of transporting biological samples, extending a doctor's eyes and ears into remote areas via video chat, and even helping deliver food, medicine, and care to patients in their homes. But before drones can become commonplace in health care, they must be safely integrated into the airspace and proved to operate without causing accidents and other problems. Even if that is accomplished, the flying robots must be accepted by both medical staff and patients, many of whom associate drones only with warfare. "When we say the word 'drones,' people think of things that fly over their heads and kill their children," says Amukele. "That's not what we're talking about here. We're talking about small, unmanned flying systems." If people become more comfortable with drones, the result could be faster, cheaper medical care. "People are starting to realize that drones can be used for good," Amukele says. "Already, in the United States, they are being used for agriculture and film making, but what they haven't been used for is healthcare. Healthcare is the industry where we need this capacity."[51]

CHAPTER 4

Medical Evacuations

Drones are being used to provide medications and other supplies for treatment in remote clinics and even in patients' homes. Sometimes such care is not enough. For patients in critical condition, their only chance for survival is to be treated in a hospital. Usually, injured or seriously ill patients are taken to hospitals by ground ambulances or medical evacuation helicopters. Some engineers believe that drones can be used for medical evacuations as well.

Medical evacuations are especially difficult in combat zones, where ground transports and helicopters have limited access, and this is one of the first planned uses of evacuation drones. Casualty evacuation is known as CASEVAC. It refers to removing an injured soldier without providing medical care in flight. It differs from medical evacuation, or MEDEVAC, in which care is provided in flight.

The Marine Corps is the first branch of the US military to pursue the use of drones to evacuate casualties from the battlefield. The Marine Corps Warfighting Laboratory (MCWL) conducted several demonstrations in 2009 and 2010 to study the feasibility of using unmanned aerial systems (UAS), or drones, for CASEVAC, as well as for transporting supplies to the front lines. These vehicles have rotors, meaning they operate more like a helicopter than an airplane. The first MCWL demonstration took place in May 2009. In this test, a Boeing Unmanned Little Bird UAS delivered water and food to a target and then evacuated a weighted mannequin, simulating a casualty. The Little Bird is a small helicopter that was outfitted with two outboard cargo pods, one on each side of the aircraft. The weighted mannequin was carried in one of the cargo pods. The flights were successful, leading to a new round of testing.

The next demonstration took place in January 2010 at the Dugway Proving Ground in Utah. This test involved the Kaman/Lockheed Martin K-Max UAS, another unmanned helicopter, which used a sling to carry cargo and the simulated casualty. The Kaman drone successfully took off and landed using its own computers. It also was tested when operated by remote pilots. The third and final demonstration took place in March 2010, also at Dugway. It also involved a helicopter-like drone, the Boeing A160 Hummingbird UAS. This test was also a success. In 2011 the US Marine Corps deployed the K-Max UAS system in Afghanistan. However, it used the drone only to move cargo, not to evacuate casualties. The drone was not yet deemed safe enough to carry human beings.

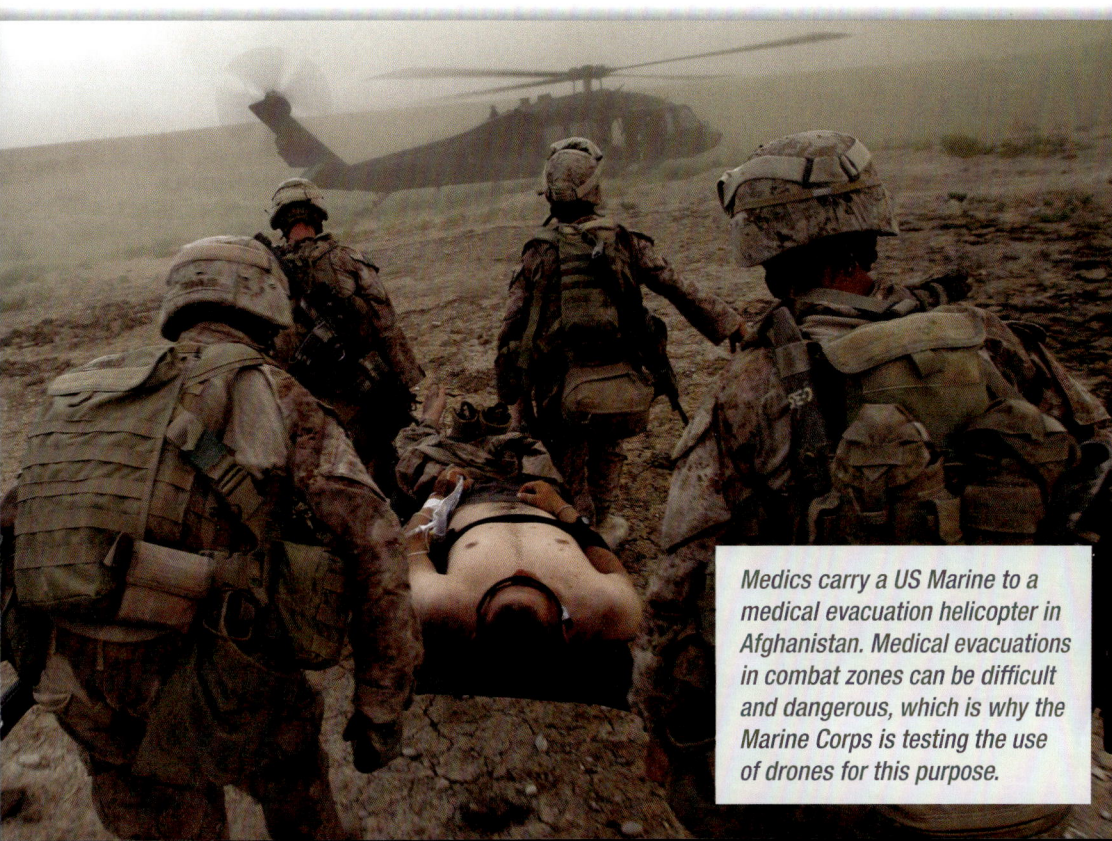

Medics carry a US Marine to a medical evacuation helicopter in Afghanistan. Medical evacuations in combat zones can be difficult and dangerous, which is why the Marine Corps is testing the use of drones for this purpose.

The Dragonfly Medical Drone

After the 2010 projects were complete, the MCWL joined with the Air Force Research Laboratory and the US Army's Telemedicine and Advanced Technology Research Center (TATRC) at Fort Detrick in Maryland to conduct further research on casualty evacuation by drone. In 2017 researchers from the TATRC revealed their plans for using a new helicopter-like drone for unmanned resupply and medical evacuation. Built by Dragonfly Pictures, which has been designing and building unmanned helicopters since 1992, the DP-14 Heavy Fuel Tandem Helicopter can execute a vertical takeoff and landing and carry a 450-pound (204 kg) payload 100 miles (161 km). Unlike the three helicopter drones tested in 2009 and 2010, the DP-14 has two external rotors, one in front and one in back. This is known as a tandem-rotor configuration.

A tandem-rotor helicopter, such as the famous Boeing CH-47 Chinook military helicopter, has a larger center of gravity than a single-rotor helicopter, making it ideal for transporting cargo. A tandem-rotor helicopter is also stable in the air, due to the fact that the two rotors turn in opposite directions, canceling out the turning force, or torque, that a single rotor has on the body of the helicopter. (Single-rotor helicopters use a small propeller located on the craft's tail to counteract the rotor's torque.) The DP-14's rotors are not very large, however, so the drone can still take off and land in areas where standard helicopters cannot go.

Researchers at the TATRC are working on how to monitor the DP-14 to determine what conditions might be like inside the drone if a patient were to ride inside it. Army researchers are measuring factors like vibration, noise, temperature, pressure, acceleration, and pitch of the aircraft. They are comparing the results to similar tests being run on UH-60 Black Hawk helicopters, which the military already uses for medical evacuations. They want to make sure that the drone is at

torque
A twisting or turning force that tends to cause rotation around an axis

NATO Standards for Unmanned Medical Evacuation

In December 2012 the NATO Technical Panel published a guide to using drones to evacuate casualties from the battlefield. The panel concluded that the use of drones for this purpose is "ethically, legally, clinically, and operationally permissible, so long as the relative risk to the casualty is not increased." NATO said four criteria must be met before a casualty can be evacuated by drone:

- The aircraft must meet all the same safety-of-flight requirements as do current manned rotary wing aircraft (helicopters).
- Environmental standards in the casualty compartment (noise, vibration, acceleration factors, air quality) must meet current standards.
- Some provision must be made to strap the patient into the drone.
- Carriage of the casualty must be internal to the aircraft.

In 2014 Urban Aeronautics' Cormorant became the first drone to be recognized by NATO for meeting its unmanned medical evacuation requirements.

Quoted in James C. Rosser et al., "Surgical and Medical Applications of Drones: A Comprehensive Review," *Journal of the Society of Laparoendoscopic Surgeons*, July–September 2018. www.ncbi.nlm.nih.gov.

---

least as safe as the helicopters in use now. The researchers are also developing a patient-support system that will transmit patient data to medics on the ground, so they can monitor the patient en route to the hospital.

Nathan Fisher, an engineer with the TATRC, says that the ideal scenario for casualty evacuation is to use a helicopter equipped with medical gear and staffed with a medical crew that can take care of a patient while flying. "That's always plan A," says Fisher. But if a helicopter cannot reach a location, a drone might be the solution. "I like to call it a plan B," says Fisher. "It's a situation where you can't get a medevac there in time, or there's no medevac assets available due to the threat situation or due to the fact that they are just at capacity."[52]

The Coming of the Cormorant

US companies are not the only ones exploring the concept of casualty evacuation by drone. Urban Aeronautics, an Israeli tech company, has also developed a drone for delivering medical supplies to a battlefield and evacuating victims from it. But the Urban Aeronautics drone, originally called the Air Mule but now known as the Cormorant, is different from the drones the US military has tested. It is not a miniature helicopter. Instead, it is powered by two internally mounted propellers, known as ducted fans.

A ducted fan is a type of propeller, or fan, that is mounted inside a cylinder, or duct. This arrangement confines the airflow created by the propeller to the space inside the cylinder. Normally, with an open propeller, some of the propeller's thrust is lost from the tips of the propeller blades. A ducted fan reduces that loss. As a result, a ducted fan generates more power than an open propeller of the same size. The engines on commercial airliners, for example, use ducted fans for maximum power.

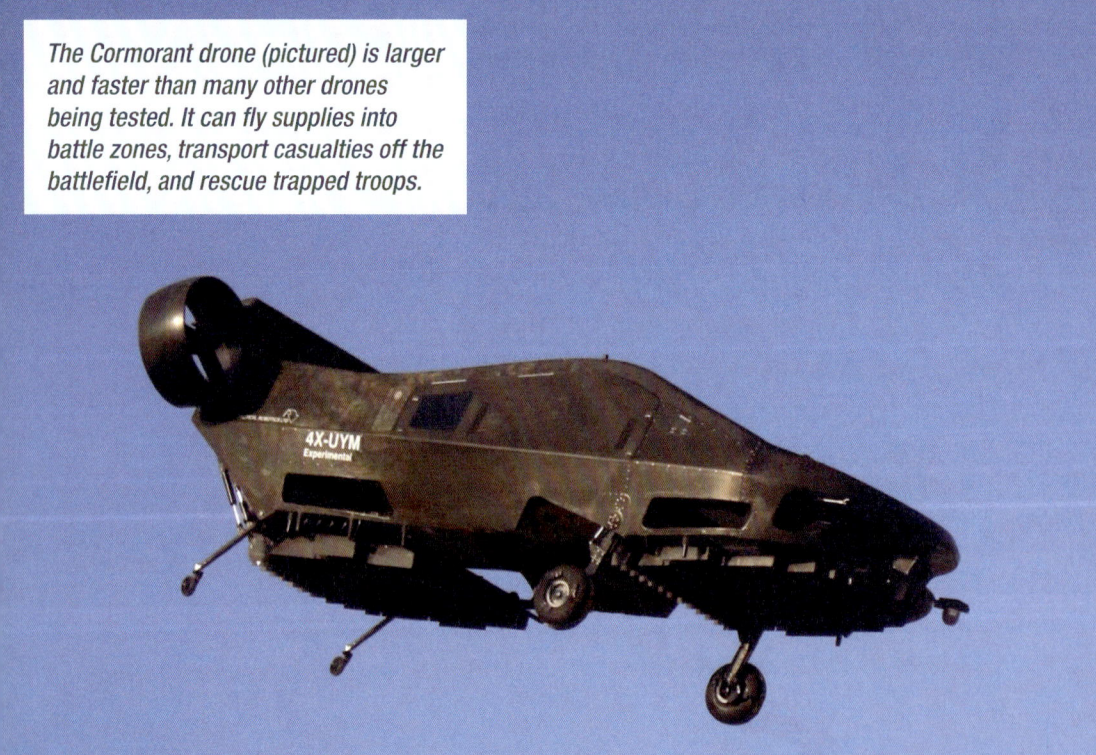

The Cormorant drone (pictured) is larger and faster than many other drones being tested. It can fly supplies into battle zones, transport casualties off the battlefield, and rescue trapped troops.

The Cormorant's ducted fans allow the car-sized vehicle to fly in very tight quarters. Since it does not have exposed rotor blades, the Cormorant can slip between buildings and pass near power lines without the risk of striking them. It is also quieter than a helicopter, because the cylindrical ducts that house the propellers muffle their sound.

Measuring 20 feet (6.2 m) long and 7.5 feet (2.3 m) tall, the Cormorant can take off vertically, like a helicopter, and carry up to 1,100 pounds (499 kg). Its top speed can reach 115 miles per hour (185 kph). With these capabilities, the Cormorant has many uses. It can fly supplies to the front lines. It can transport casualties off the battlefield. And it can be used to rescue healthy troops holed up in a defensive position or behind enemy lines. Rafi Yoeli, CEO of Urban Aeronautics, says:

> [It could fly to] anyone out in the field who needs water, food, batteries, supplies, medical equipment and so forth. Later, it could be used to fetch soldiers that you don't want to leave behind or are wounded. There are plenty of situations where you cannot send a helicopter—for example, in the middle of fighting where you want to evacuate people from a street or from a narrow roof.[53]

Yoeli says the idea for building a vehicle that can go where helicopters cannot was born out of the 2006 Israel-Hezbollah war, some of which was fought in Hezbollah-dominated neighborhoods in southern Beirut, Lebanon. Because of the conflict's urban setting, it took an average of five and a half hours to evacuate wounded Israeli soldiers. "One reason is the ground-to-air fire," Yoeli says. "The other is because of the physical limitations of a helicopter's rotor, it cannot land in a mountainous or obstacle area."[54] What was needed, Yoeli believed, was a small, flying rescue vehicle that did not have a helicopter's large rotors.

Updating the Flying Jeep

Yoeli's vision of an evacuation drone was inspired in part by the successful tests of the US Army's VZ-8P aircraft, a type of flying jeep built for the US government by the Piasecki Aircraft company in the 1950s. Yoeli took the VZ-8P's successful test flights as proof that a drone large enough to carry a human being was feasible. His team of engineers borrowed the VZ-8P's design of having two wide-diameter ducted fans in the front and back of the aircraft. The engineers combined the two-fan design with modern materials, including computer components and lightweight carbon fiber composite material to make the drone's fuselage. Altogether, Urban Aeronautics has patented thirty-nine separate inventions that went into the Cormorant's design.

Like hybrid electric cars, the Cormorant uses a combination of gasoline and electricity to power the craft. The drone is equipped with two powerful gas turbine engines, one on each side of the patient's cabin. The gas engines drive an electric generator. The generator powers the electric motors in the large ducted fans. It also powers the two rear-mounted drive fans that provide stability and forward thrust.

In February 2019 Urban Aeronautics held a demonstration at the Megiddo Airfield in northern Israel to show the Cormorant's ability to carry out medical evacuation missions in combat zones. The demonstration included taking off with a load of simulated medical cargo, flying to a specified point of delivery, and off-loading the cargo. The demonstration staff then loaded the drone with a medical training mannequin, simulating an injured soldier. With the simulated patient aboard, the drone returned to its point of origin. Except for the off-loading of the cargo and the loading of the "casualty" into the drone, the entire mission was per-

gas turbine

A type of internal combustion engine in which burning of an air-fuel mixture produces hot gases that spin a turbine to produce power

The Piasecki Flying Jeep

Urban Aeronautics' Cormorant evacuation drone is modeled after the US Army's VZ-8P aircraft, a small rotorcraft built by Piasecki Aircraft in the 1950s. Also known as the Piasecki Airgeep, the VZ-8P was a manned vehicle capable of flying two people. It was equipped with two large-diameter ducted fans, one in front and one in back. The VZ-8P's ducted fans allowed the aircraft to take off vertically to gain altitude. They also provided forward thrust when the nose of the flying jeep was tilted down, with the ducted fans pushing it forward from underneath and behind.

The VZ-P8 was also tested by the US Navy. Outfitted with floats so it could set down on the water, it was known by the navy as the Model 59N. The idea was to use it to travel from ship to ship or ship to shore, or even to rescue sailors in the water.

The Piasecki Airgeep could reach an altitude of 3,000 feet (914 m) and cruise at 70 miles per hour (113 kph), meeting the military's specifications. However, not foreseeing future involvement in urban warfare, such as the wars in Afghanistan and Iraq, the government decided against deploying the flying jeeps.

---

formed automatically by the drone. "It could revolutionize several aspects of warfare, including medical evacuation of soldiers on the battlefield,"[55] says Tal Inbar, head of the UAV research center at Israel's Fisher Institute for Air and Space Strategic Studies.

The Cormorant is equipped with an onboard patient monitor. The monitor transmits vital information about the condition of the patient to the crew on the ground. The interior of the Cormorant is also outfitted with a video camera for two-way communication with the patient throughout the flight.

The US Army is looking at using the Cormorant for medical evacuations and for transporting supplies. However, to convince the US Department of Defense that the Cormorant is worth its hefty $14 million price tag, Urban Aeronautics must prove the vehicle's durability. "When you supply a vehicle to the customer, you need to offer them a guarantee that it will work for 500 hours or 1,000 hours or so many take-offs and landings," says Yoeli. "So, we need to develop the knowledge of the lifespan of the components and maybe redesign some of them."[56]

The Cormorant is the only drone recognized by the North Atlantic Treaty Organization (NATO), a joint American-European military defense organization, to meet its strict standards for transporting human beings. It also meets the organization's requirements for delivering cargo. The certification means the craft is ideal as a medical drone that is capable of carrying medical supplies and evacuating patients. The drone has also been designed in accordance with FAA passenger-carrying certification standards. This means it could be certified to transport civilians as well.

Civilian Applications

The Cormorant holds great promise for civilians. It could be used in place of a traditional emergency response vehicle or MEDEVAC helicopter to transport people seriously injured in a traffic accident, especially in an area with traffic congestion or where MEDEVAC helicopters cannot go. "There's the concept of the golden hour," says Philip Werthman, a US-based adviser to the board of Urban Aeronautics. "In order to maximize survivability in an accident, you need to get to the victims and get that victim evacuated within an hour."[57] Motor vehicle accidents are the second-highest cause of accidental death in the United States, according to the Centers for Disease Control and Prevention, with about thirty-seven thousand fatalities a year. Even a small increase in the survival rate of traffic accident victims could save hundreds if not thousands of lives a year in the United State alone.

A person-carrying drone has rescue potential as well. For example, it could be sent to rescue hikers stranded in rocky or wooded terrain where a helicopter could not land. It could airlift people to safety from their rooftops during floods and hurricanes, where power lines, trees, and other obstructions might prevent

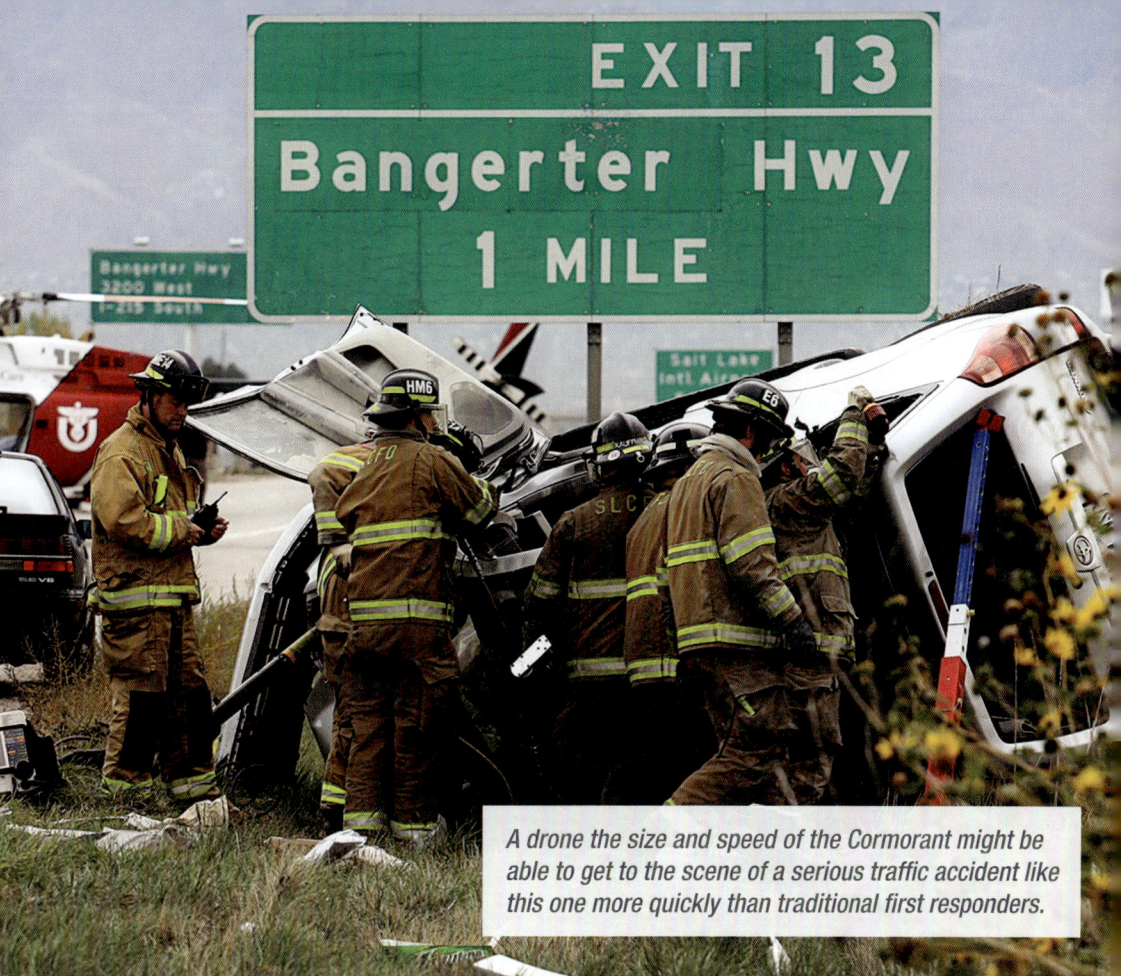

A drone the size and speed of the Cormorant might be able to get to the scene of a serious traffic accident like this one more quickly than traditional first responders.

helicopters from going. It could also remove civilians from dangerous situations such as an area contaminated with radiation. "Just imagine a dirty bomb in a city and chemical substance of something else and this vehicle can come in robotically, remotely piloted, come into a street,"[58] says Yoeli.

Evacuation drones do present risks. A crash could well be fatal for the people being moved. In addition, they pose a danger to people under their flight paths. If a small drone carrying a payload of less than 50 pounds (22.7 kg) falls from the sky, the damage on the ground

dirty bomb

A type of nuclear weapon that uses radioactive nuclear waste material and conventional explosives to spread radiation through a targeted area

51

would be slight, unless it hits a person directly. However, the Cormorant weighs 1,700 pounds (771 kg) empty and 3,100 pounds (1,406 kg) fully loaded. "A vehicle this size obviously brings very significant safety issues,"[59] says Ravi Vaidyanathan, a drone expert at Imperial College London. If a Cormorant crashed into a building or onto a street with heavy traffic, the results could be catastrophic. The Cormorant has been outfitted with a parachute that would bring the drone to earth safely in the event of a catastrophic engine failure. However, the parachute's deployment and reliability must be proved with extensive testing.

Medical evacuation drones can save lives both on the battlefield and in everyday life. According to the US Army Medical Research and Materiel Command, helicopter medical evacuations have made a tremendous contribution to casualty survival, which is at the highest level in military history. The survival rates of US casualties in Afghanistan and Iraq were 89.9 percent, compared to 69.7 percent in World War II. Similarly, civilian MEDEVAC helicopters and emergency response vehicles have saved countless lives by getting patients to hospitals within the "golden hour," when medical attention is most effective. The deployment of evacuation drones to places MEDEVAC helicopters and emergency vehicles cannot reach could raise that survival rate even higher. A worldwide network of medical evacuation drones could, for the first time in history, bring first-rate emergency medical services within reach of every person on the planet.

SOURCE NOTES

Introduction: A New Era in Medical Care
1. Quoted in Sigal Samuel, "Ghana's New Lifesaving Drones: Like Uber, but for Blood," *Vox*, June 4, 2019. www.vox.com.
2. Quoted in Andrew Nusca, "The Trick to Achieving Universal Health Care? Drones," *Fortune*, April 2, 2019. https://fortune.com.
3. Quoted in David Freeman, "A Drone Just Flew a Kidney to a Transplant Patient for the First Time Ever. It Won't Be the Last," NBC News, May 3, 2019. www.nbcnews.com.
4. Manohari Balasingam, "Drones in Medicine—the Rise of the Machines," *International Journal of Clinical Practice*, August 29, 2017. https://onlinelibrary.wiley.com.

Chapter 1: Transporting Organs for Transplants
5. Quoted in Karen Zraick, "Like 'Uber for Organs': Drone Delivers Kidney to Maryland Woman," *New York Times*, April 30, 2019. www.nytimes.com.
6. Quoted in Bill Seiler, "University of Maryland's Schools of Medicine and Engineering First to Use Unmanned Aircraft to Successfully Deliver Kidney for Transplant at University of Maryland Medical Center," University of Maryland Medical Center, April 26, 2019. www.umms.org.
7. Quoted in Ann W. Schmidt, "Drone Delivers Kidney for Transplant in Maryland, Doctors Say: 'It's a First Step,'" Fox News, April 29, 2019. www.foxnews.com.
8. Quoted in Zraick, "Like 'Uber for Organs.'"
9. Quoted in Schmidt, "Drone Delivers Kidney for Transplant in Maryland."
10. Quoted in Seiler, "University of Maryland's Schools of Medicine and Engineering First to Use Unmanned Aircraft to Successfully Deliver Kidney for Transplant at University of Maryland Medical Center."

11. Quoted in Seiler, "University of Maryland's Schools of Medicine and Engineering First to Use Unmanned Aircraft to Successfully Deliver Kidney for Transplant at University of Maryland Medical Center."
12. Quoted in Zraick, "Like 'Uber for Organs.'"
13. Quoted in Oliver Luft, "Why Drones Are Set to Disrupt the Medical Industry—and Help Save Lives," *HERE 360* (blog), June 5, 2019. https://360.here.com.
14. Quoted in Freeman, "A Drone Just Flew a Kidney to a Transplant Patient for the First Time Ever."
15. Quoted in Zraick, "Like 'Uber for Organs.'"
16. Quoted in Seiler, "University of Maryland's Schools of Medicine and Engineering First to Use Unmanned Aircraft to Successfully Deliver Kidney for Transplant at University of Maryland Medical Center."
17. Quoted in Seiler, "University of Maryland's Schools of Medicine and Engineering First to Use Unmanned Aircraft to Successfully Deliver Kidney for Transplant at University of Maryland Medical Center."
18. Quoted in Zraick, "Like 'Uber for Organs.'"
19. Quoted in Freeman, "A Drone Just Flew a Kidney to a Transplant Patient for the First Time Ever."
20. Quoted in Freeman, "A Drone Just Flew a Kidney to a Transplant Patient for the First Time Ever."
21. Quoted in Seiler, "University of Maryland's Schools of Medicine and Engineering First to Use Unmanned Aircraft to Successfully Deliver Kidney for Transplant at University of Maryland Medical Center."

Chapter 2: Delivering Medical Supplies

22. Quoted in Chloe Taylor, "Drones Deliver Vaccines to One-Month Old Baby in Remote Island of Vanuatu," CNBC, December 19, 2018. www.cnbc.com.
23. Quoted in Renee Knight, "Drones Deliver Healthcare," Inside Unmanned Systems, September 3, 2016. http://insideunmannedsystems.com.
24. Quoted in Will Yacowicz, "Robots to the Rescue: Blood Delivery via Drone Is Coming to U.S.," Inc.com, August 3, 2016. www.inc.com.

25. Quoted in Evan Ackerman and Michael Koziol, "In the Air with Zipline's Medical Delivery Drones," *IEEE Spectrum*, April 30, 2019. https://spectrum.ieee.org.
26. Quoted in Ackerman and Koziol, "In the Air with Zipline's Medical Delivery Drones."
27. Quoted in Ackerman and Koziol, "In the Air with Zipline's Medical Delivery Drones."
28. Quoted in Knight, "Drones Deliver Healthcare."
29. Quoted in Samuel, "Ghana's New Lifesaving Drones."
30. Quoted in Samuel, "Ghana's New Lifesaving Drones."
31. Quoted in Jake Bright, "Drone Delivery Startup Zipline Launches UAV Medical Program in Ghana," TechCrunch, May 4, 2019. https://techcrunch.com.
32. Quoted in Knight, "Drones Deliver Healthcare."
33. Quoted in EMS World, "Nev. City Receives FAA Approval for Drone Delivery of AEDs," March 8, 2019. www.emsworld.com.
34. Quoted in Knight, "Drones Deliver Healthcare."
35. Jeremy Tucker, "A Role for Drones in Healthcare," Fierce Healthcare, December 10, 2013. www.fiercehealthcare.com.
36. Quoted in Knight, "Drones Deliver Healthcare."

Chapter 3: Remote Testing and Care

37. Quoted in CBS News, "First-of-Its-Kind Drone Program in North Carolina Is Helping Diagnose Patients Faster," May 7, 2019. www.cbsnews.com.
38. Quoted in CBS News, "First-of-Its-Kind Drone Program in North Carolina Is Helping Diagnose Patients Faster."
39. Quoted in Samantha Bresnahan, "The Good Drones: Air Delivery of Blood Samples Could Save Lives," CNN, February 19, 2016. https://edition.cnn.com.
40. Quoted in Yacowicz, "Robots to the Rescue."
41. Quoted in Bresnahan, "The Good Drones."
42. Quoted in Steven Ashley, "One of These Drones Could Save Your Life," NBC News, January 12, 2017. www.nbcnews.com.
43. Quoted in Ashley, "One of These Drones Could Save Your Life."
44. Quoted in Ashley, "One of These Drones Could Save Your Life."
45. Quoted in Ashley, "One of These Drones Could Save Your Life."

46. Quoted in David Robertson, "Bibbidi Bobbidi Bots: ASPIRE to Improve Lives of Senior Citizens," Coordinated Science Laboratory, August 13, 2015. https://csl.illinois.edu.
47. Quoted in Knight, "Drones Deliver Healthcare."
48. Quoted in Robertson, "Bibbidi Bobbidi Bots."
49. Quoted in Pauline Canteneur, "Autonomous Drones Soon Assisting Elderly People in the Home?," Atelier US, October 13, 2016. https://atelier.bnpparibas.
50. Quoted in Knight, "Drones Deliver Healthcare."
51. Quoted in Bresnahan, "The Good Drones."

Chapter 4: Medical Evacuations

52. Quoted in C. Todd Lopez, "Army Looking into Unmanned Medevac, Medical Resupply," US Army, October 13, 2017. www.army.mil.
53. Quoted in Leo Kelion, "AirMule Military Drone Set to Dodge Trees in Tests," BBC, January 14, 2016. www.bbc.com.
54. Quoted in Jonathan Hunt, "Self-Flying Vehicle Could Come to US by 2022," Fox News, June 1, 2018. www.foxnews.com.
55. Quoted in Elana Ringler, "Israel's 'Flying Car' Passenger Drone Moves Closer to Delivery," Reuters, January 4, 2017. www.reuters.com.
56. Quoted in Kelion, "AirMule Military Drone Set to Dodge Trees in Tests."
57. Quoted in Ringler, "Israel's 'Flying Car' Passenger Drone Moves Closer to Delivery."
58. Quoted in Ringler, "Israel's 'Flying Car' Passenger Drone Moves Closer to Delivery."
59. Quoted in Kelion, "AirMule Military Drone Set to Dodge Trees in Tests."

FOR FURTHER RESEARCH

Books

Michael J. Boyle, *The Drone Age*. New York: Oxford, 2020.

Alex Elliott, *Inside Drones*. New York: Rosen, 2019.

John L. Hakala, *How Drones Will Impact Society*. San Diego: ReferencePoint, 2018.

Kathryn Hulick, *How Robotics Is Changing the World*. San Diego: ReferencePoint, 2019.

Stuart A. Kallen, *What Is the Future of Drones?* San Diego: ReferencePoint, 2017.

Internet Sources

Evan Ackerman and Michael Koziol, "In the Air with Zipline's Medical Delivery Drones," *IEEE Spectrum*, April 30, 2019. https://spectrum.ieee.org.

Steven Ashley, "One of These Drones Could Save Your Life," NBC News, January 12, 2017. www.nbcnews.com.

Renee Knight, "Drones Deliver Healthcare," Inside Unmanned Systems, September 3, 2016. http://insideunmannedsystems.com.

James C. Rosser et al., "Surgical and Medical Applications of Drones: A Comprehensive Review," *Journal of the Society of Laparoendoscopic Surgeons*, July–September 2018. www.ncbi.nlm.nih.gov.

Tammy Waitt, "Self-Flying War Vehicle Coming to the USA," American Security Today, June 3, 2018. https://americansecuritytoday.com.

Websites

Center for the Study of the Drone (http://dronecenter.bard.edu). A publication of Bard College, this website features a weekly roundup of news about drones, including fixed wing, commercial, and military drones. It includes interviews with leaders in the drone industry from government, business, and the arts.

Drones in Healthcare (www.dronesinhealthcare.com). This blog provides a roundup of the latest news on the medical application of drones. It includes exclusive interviews with medical drone experts and links to relevant videos.

DroneLife (www.dronelife.com). This blog has up-to-date news and information about drone products, regulations, and business. It includes a section devoted to drone videos and another to podcasts. The blog also includes separate sections for specific industries, including agriculture, mining, police and fire, delivery, real estate, surveying, inspection, and construction.

sUAS News (www.suasnews.com). Founded by drone pilots and professionals, sUAS News is the leading news and information source for unmanned aviation. This website includes a searchable drone safety map, color coded to indicate flying hazards, including airports, ground hazards, and legal restrictions.

INDEX

Note: Boldface page numbers indicate illustrations.

Ackerman, Evan, 22
Africa, Zipline International in, 4–6, **5**, 20–25, **21**
AirBox, 34
Air Force Research Laboratory, 44–45
Airgeep, 48, 49
Air Mule. *See* Urban Aeronautics' Cormorant
Akufo-Addo, Nana, 25
Alexander, Charlie, 10, 14
altitude, defined, 4
Amukele, Timothy, 33, 35, 41
automated external defibrillators (AEDs), **25**, 25–27

Balasingam, Manohari, 7
Bimpe, Israel, 21–22
Black Hawk helicopters, 44
blood and blood products
  in Ghana, 24
  ordering and delivery of, 21–22
  shelf life of, 20
Boadu, George Appiah, 24
Boeing CH-47 Chinook helicopters, 44
Boeing Unmanned Little Bird UAS tests, 42–43
Brock, Stan, 28

cardiac arrest, 26–27
casualty evacuations (CASEVACs), 42–43, **46**
CH-47 Chinook helicopters, 44
Core Laboratory (Johns Hopkins Hospital) test, 34–35
Cormorant. *See* Urban Aeronautics' Cormorant
costs
  compared to using helicopters, 19–20
  cutting health care, 40–41
  delivery of organs for transplants, 16
  government subsidies, 22–23
  opposition to drone use and, 24–25
  payloads and, 22–23
  reductions in blood waste, 20–21
  Urban Aeronautics' Cormorant, 49–50
  WakeMed Hospital program revenue, 31

defibrillators, **25**, 25–27
dialysis, kidney, 8
dirty bombs, defined, 51
DP-14 Heavy Fuel Tandem Helicopter, 44–45
Dragonfly Pictures, 44
drones
  dangers of using, 51–52
  defined, 4
  types of, 4, 44
ducted fans, 46–47, 48

elderly, in-home care for, 38–40

Federal Aviation Administration (FAA)
  experimental program of drone delivery flights beyond visual line of sight, 27
  flying regulations for small unmanned aircraft, 17
  custom drones and, 12
  operation within pilot's line of sight, 13, 16, 38
  passenger-carrying certification standards, 50
  restrictions on privately owned drones, 37–38
Field Innovation Team, 33
Fisher, Nathan, 45
fixed-wing drones
  capturing, 26

59

described, 4
   launching described, 22
Flirtey, **25**, 27, 28, **29**, 33
flying jeeps, 48, 49
Fore, Henrietta H., 19

gas turbines, defined, 48
Ghana, 4, 5, 24–25
Ginn, Stuart, 32
Glispy, Trina, 8, 10–12
Global Positioning System (GPS) data, 6
Google Glass, 36–37
Graboyes, Robert, 6, 17

Head, Mark, 25–26
head-tracking software, defined, 39
Health and Medicine Division (HMD) of the National Academies of Sciences, Engineering and Medicine, 26
helicopters
   Boeing CH-47 Chinook helicopters, 44
   compared to Urban Aeronautics' Cormorant, 47
   costs, compared to using drones, 19–20
   DP-14 Heavy Fuel Tandem Helicopter, 44–45
   UH-60 Black Hawk helicopters, 44
Hinds Community College, 37
Hovakimyan, Naira, 38, 39–40
Human Organ Monitoring and Quality Assurance Apparatus for Long-Distance Travel (HOMAL), 12–14

Inbar, Tal, 49
indoor uses, 7
   in-home care, 38–40
   as pharmacy porters, 29–30
infrared, defined, 37

Johns Hopkins University School of Medicine, 33

Kaman/Lockheed Martin K-Max UAS, 43
kidney disease and dialysis, 8

kidney transplants, 8–12, **9**
K-Max UAS system, 43
Koziol, Michael, 22

Ledgard, Jonathan, 22–23
Let's Fly Wisely, 28, **29**
Little Bird UAS tests, 42–43
Lott, Dennis, 38

malaria, 24
Malawi, 6
Marine Corps Warfighting Laboratory (MCWL), 42–45
Marsh, Christopher, 16
MasterFlight, 27
maternal mortality, 20
Matternet, 7, 31–32
medical equipment delivery, **25**, 25–27
medical evacuations (MEDEVACs)
   battlefield survival rates and, 52
   versus casualty evacuations, 42
   in combat zones, **43**
   NATO standards, 45, 50
   UH-60 Black Hawk helicopters for, 44
   Urban Aeronautics' Cormorant, **46**
      advantages, 47, 50
      medical equipment on board, 49
      multiple uses of, 50–51, **51**
      safety issues, 52
      standards met by, 45, 50
      test demonstration, 48–49
medical samples and supplies delivery
   in Africa, 4, **5**, 5–6, 20–21
   cost factors, 19, 20–21
   described, 21–22
   by drones compared to motorbikes, 22
   government subsidies for, 22–23
   reduction in waste and, 20–21
   in US, 7
   vaccines, medications, and blood supplies, 23–24
medicine delivery, 7, 23, 34
Mid-Atlantic Aviation Partnership (Virginia Tech), 28
Model 59N (US Navy), 49

motorbikes, current payload capacity, 22

National Academies of Sciences, Engineering, and Medicine, 26–27
National Aeronautics and Space Administration (NASA), 28
"nests," 20
New York Times (newspaper), 11
NICER (Non-Intrusive Cooperative Empathetic Robots), 40
noncommunicable diseases, worldwide annual deaths from, 33
North Atlantic Treaty Organization (NATO), standards for unmanned medical evacuations, 45, 50
Nowai, Joy, 19

Oksenhorn, Ryan, 19–20
organ transplants, delivery of, 7
  cost factor, 16
  effect of quicker organ deliveries, 15–16
  kidneys, 8–12, **9**
  in less developed countries, 18
  maintaining organ viability, 10, 11, 13, 15, 18
  monitoring of condition of organ during, 13–14
  obstacles to drone deliveries, 16–17
  shortage of organs for, 9–10
  transportation options, 14–15

Papua New Guinea, 6
Pargoe, Brandon, 34
payload, defined, 12
payloads
  capacity of motorbikes, 22
  financial viability and, 22–23
  potential future, 16, 27
  Zipline drones, 22, 23
pharmacy porters, 29–30
Piasecki Aircraft VZ-8P Airgeep, 48, 49
Pines, Darryll J., 18
pneumatic tubes, defined, 30
Pucciarella, Anthony, 12

RAM, 25, 27

redundancy, defined, 12
Reno, Nevada, **25**, 27
Rinaudo, Keller, 6, 20, 33
rotorcrafts
  drones as, 4
  landing, 26
  tandem-rotor configuration, 44
  unmanned aerial systems, 42
Rwanda, **5**, 5–6, 20–24, **21**

safety
  backup systems, 12
  deliveries in urban areas, 34–35
  features on next generation of Zipline drones, 23
  indoor drones and, 39
  lockbox technology for medicines, 34
  need for reliable communications and collision avoidance systems, 17, **18**, 38
  operation within pilot's line of sight, 13, 16, 27, 38
  of people under flight paths, 51–52
  WakeMed Hospital program as experiment, 32
Scalea, Joseph, **14**
  on future drone speeds and payloads, 16
  HOMAL test, 12
  on organ transplants
    effect of drone technology on, 11–12
    effect of long transportation times, 15
    effect of quicker deliveries, 15–16
    long-range delivery of, 15
    monitoring of condition of, during flights, 13–14
Schieve, Hillary, 27
speed
  cardiac patient survival and, 26
  compared to other transport methods, 31–32
  disease diagnoses and, 4, 33
  effect of on organ deliveries, 15–16
  FAA rules for maximum, for small unmanned aircraft, 17

future drone payloads and, 16
medicine delivery and, 7, 23
organ deliveries and, 10, 11, 13, 15, 18
Stavanja, Will, 30
Strege, Dennis, 27
Subbarao, Italo, 35–36, 37
Swiss Post, 7
Switzerland, 7
Swoop Aero, 6

tandem-rotor configuration, 44
telemedicine
defined, 35
drones being built for, 37
equipment needed for, 35–36, **36**, 37
examples of, 35, 36–37
Telemedicine and Advanced Technology Research Center (TATRC), 44–45
testing remotely, examples of samples collected for, 31
Tissandier, Frédérique, 24
torque, defined, 44
transponder, defined, 23
Tucker, Jeremy, 30, 40–41

UH-60 Black Hawk helicopters, 44
United Network for Organ Sharing (UNOS), 9–10
United Parcel Service (UPS), 7, 31–32
United States, Zipline International in, 7
University of Illinois at Urbana-Champaign, 38–39
unmanned aerial systems (UASs), 42
unmanned aerial vehicles (UAVs), 4
Unmanned Little Bird UAS tests, 42–43
Urban Aeronautics' Cormorant, **46**
advantages, 47, 50, **51**

cost, 49–50
ducted fans for powering, 46–47, 48
inspiration for, 48, 49
medical equipment on board, 49
multiple uses of, 50–51, **51**
safety issues, 52
standards met by, 45, 50
test demonstration, 48–49
urban environments
advantages of Cormorant in, 47, 50, **51**
deliveries in, 34–35
US Army's Telemedicine and Advanced Technology Research Center (TATRC), 44–45
US Army's VZ-8P aircraft, 48, 49
US Navy's Model 59N, 49

vaccines, delivery in remote areas, 23–24
Vaidyanathan, Ravi, 52
Vanuatu, 6, 19
Virginia Tech, 28
VZ-8P aircraft (US Army), 48, 49

WakeMed Hospital program, 7, 31–32
Werthman, Philip, 50
Wiredu, Kobena, 4
World Health Organization, 24, 33

Yoeli, Rafi, 47, 48, 50, 51

Zipline International
in Africa, 4–6, **5**, 20–25, **21**
current payload capacity, 22
in Pacific island nations, 6
payload of next generation of drones, 23
in US, 7

PICTURE CREDITS

Cover: sarawuth702/iStock

 5: Kristin Palitza/picture-alliance/Newscom
 9: crystal light/Shutterstock
14: krtphotoslive/TNS/Newscom
18: Associated Press
21: Kristin Palitza/picture-alliance/Newscom
25: Associated Press
29: Associated Press
32: angellodeco/Shutterstock
36: Associated Press
40: Photographee.eu/Shutterstock
43: Associated Press
46: Tactical Robotics/Newscom
51: Rich Legg/iStock

ABOUT THE AUTHOR

Bradley Steffens is a poet, a novelist, and an award-winning author of more than fifty nonfiction books for children and young adults.